Child-led Tube-management and Tube-weaning

Marguerite Dunitz-Scheer · Peter J. Scheer

Child-led Tube-management and Tube-weaning

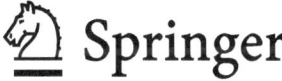 Springer

Marguerite Dunitz-Scheer
NoTube.com
Graz, Austria

Peter J. Scheer
NoTube.com
Graz, Austria

ISBN 978-3-031-09089-9   ISBN 978-3-031-09090-5   (eBook)
https://doi.org/10.1007/978-3-031-09090-5

This Springer imprint is published by the registered company Springer Nature Switzerland AG
The registered company address is: Gewerbestrasse 11, 6330 Cham, Switzerland

This book is dedicated to Jack David Dunitz (1923–2021) my beloved father and a scientist who lived through the 80s most exciting years of human science, as he often mentioned. He encouraged me to respect the very basic abilities of human nature, to observe carefully and patiently, and to trust an infant more than assumptions and interpretations.

To our children (Judith, Anna S., Anna Ch., Wolfi, Lilli, Samy, Aaron, Noah, Doris, Karim, and Jasmin), as well to our grandchildren (Mia, Rosa, Jonathan, Gavriel, Miriam, Alma, Valerie, Theresa, Fridolin, Liam, Louis, Sophia, Sandro, and Phoebe) who taught us more than anybody else during our shared lives.

Preface

This book is the result of thousands of encounters with tube-fed infants and their families over the past four decades. The ailing and fragile children suffering from a myriad of medical and nutritional conditions acted as our muses and mentors. Their parents, always steadfast, never waning in their love and support taught us more than we could have imagined. This said, this book's format is catered to the medical professional, designed and written for pediatricians, medical doctors, child surgeons, nurses, dieticians, occupational therapists, speech and language pathologists (SLPs), feeding specialists, psychologists, infant psychiatrists, early interventionists as well as any parent involved and interested with the given topic. The core subject of our work is the medically fragile child (MFC) on enteral nutrition support (ENS) by means of a feeding tube (ENT). The term ENT addresses the issue of standardized food supplementation assisted by a feeding tube. Bypassing the mouth and esophagus by means of a feeding tube involves an impact also including unintended and unpredictable effects on various physical, biochemical, sensory, functional, emotional, and social levels. Using an artificial bypass into the gut by nasogastric tube (NG), gastrostomy (PEG) or directly into the jejunal tract (JPEG) is therefore not only an exclusive selective nutritional intervention but also the cause for intended and adverse effects and externalities.

As trained pediatricians and psychotherapists, we have been treating severe eating and feeding disorders of children since the early 1980s; we have also learnt an immense amount about many different aspects regarding ENS and ENT. The growing population of tube-dependent children in the past decades—caused by the impressive progress especially in neonatal and cardiac child surgery—has encouraged us to understand even more on this issue. Frustrated children and parents urged us to seek out new therapeutic methods for the problems caused by the use or withdrawal of temporary ENT—what we term tube weaning. For this reason, we must express our gratitude to all the concerned parents and suffering children who sought our help the last 40 years. They have helped us to understand how to develop a concept apt for transitioning the child from intrusive enteral feeding to sustainable oral feeding. With the method presented here as a book of its own right for the very first time, we have weaned over 5000 children successfully and permanently off their feeding tubes. With this book we aim to pass on the knowledge we have garnered in over four decades of clinical practice to other parents and professionals. Before anything else, the art of successful tube weaning requires an individually tailored evaluation of medical, nutritional, sensory, developmental, metabolic, and growth-related findings. Furthermore, a thorough analysis of the social, emotional, and behavioral aspects of each child is also necessary to prevent any of these issues inhibiting the progress of the chosen developmental process as it progresses.

Reviewing the literature around this subject has been a source of inspiration and has provided us with critical self-reflection. In presenting our own research since years at pediatric conferences and in numerous scientific journals, we have received critical but helpful international response, from which we have learnt even more allowing us to further improve our method continuously. We advocate for a pediatrician who has led a multiprofesional team. Our main goal is to reach as many professionals as possible looking after families with a tube-fed child. Thus, we would like to offer insight, information, and our own ideas on how to approach and understand child-led tube management and tube weaning. We present our interdisciplinary method which combines peer-reviewed evidence-based scientific research with our own vast and varied experiences.

The topic itself has kept us fascinated and continues to do so up to this day.

Graz, Austria   Marguerite Dunitz-Scheer
Graz, Austria   Peter J. Scheer

Acknowledgments

We thank the Medical University Graz for its live-long support. Beat Hadorn and Ronald Kurz heads of the pediatric hospital encouraged us to start working in the field of psychosomatics. In 1986, only little was known about infants affected by eating disorders. The 1. Congress of the World Association for Infant Mental Health (WAIMH) brought the most outstanding researchers of that time and our teachers Bob Emde, Joy Osofski, and Serge Lebovici, Irene Chatoor to Austria. We are grateful that the WAIMH was inspired by that meeting to find a German-speaking branch (GAIMH). Furthermore, we were involved in the pediatric part of the Diagnostic Classification of the Zero To Three (ZTT-DC) Association in Washington, DC, and introduced its manual into German-speaking countries by translating and publishing it at Springer. The interaction with colleagues like K.-H. Brisch from Ulm and Kai v. Klitzing, Leipzig as well as the unnamed members of the GAIMH was fruitful. The acceptance of the subject by the World Association of Pediatric Gastroenterology and Nutrition and its journal (JPGN) supported the acceptance in the scientific community. Our eldest son Samy started a little firm offering online coaching for infants suffering from eating disorders in 2009, which developed under the leadership of our son Wolfi to a reasonable non-profit business employing 20 professionals such as Elisabeth Beckenbach, Eva Kerschischnik, Kessy Frenzel, Gertraud Kaltenbäck, Sabine Marinschek, Karoline Pahsini, Marion Russel, Valerie Sulzer, M. Wutsch, Aaron Scheer, and many others from whom we learned a lot by discussing different points of view. Numerous others—including students of psychotherapy—were able to learn the child-led approach hands-on in our Graz-based outpatient clinic the Eating School. We are very grateful for the final English corrections of the text, which were made by Jonathan and Lola Sichrovsky. Finally, we thank our current CEO Daniela Schachner-Blazizek who supports every step we take enthusiastically.

Contents

List of Abbreviations

ASD	Autism Spectrum Disorder
BPD	Broncho-Pulmonary Disorder
CDH	Congenital Diaphragmatic Hernia
CdLS	Cornelia de-Lange Syndrome
CP	Cerebral Palsy
DACH	Germany-Austria-Swiss
EA	Esophageal Atresia
EAT	Early Autonomy Training
ECMO	Extra-Corporal Membrane Oxygenation
ENS	Enteral Nutrition Support
ENT	Enteral Nutrition by Tube
ES	Eating School
ESPEGHAN	European Society for Paediatric Gastroenterology, Hepatology and Nutrition
FTT	Failure To Thrive
GERD	Gastrointestinal Reflux Disease
GI	Gastro-Intestinal
GMFCS	Gross Motor Function Classification System
IUGR	Intra-Uterine Growth Retardation
JPEG	Jejunal Percutaneous Feeding Tube
MFC	Medically Fragile Child
NG-tube	Naso-Gastric feeding tube
NICU	Neonatal Intensive Care Unit
NOFT	Non-Organic Failure to Thrive
PEG	Percutaneous Endoscopic Gastrostomy
PICU	Perinatal Intensive Care Unit
PPI	Proton Pump Inhibitor
PTSD	Post-Traumatic Stress Disorder
ROP	Retinopathy of Prematurity
SGA	Small for Gestational Age
SLT	Speech Language Therapist
VLBW	Very Low Birth Weight
WHO	World Health Organization

The Fascination of Intrinsic Learning Processes

Growing up in Switzerland and Austria, there was a sort of certainty that every child was able to ski or swim by the age of 3 or 4, some even seemed born already masters at both! But on visiting Holland, we saw everyone using a bicycle instead of their feet. Marguerite and I could not ride a bicycle until the age of 11 and never learnt to ice-skate at all. So, learning to ski, to swim, to ride a bike, or to ice-skate seemed to be above all technical aspects culturally defined. Later in life, both of us aided young Dutch students on ski holidays in the Alps or supported panic-stricken tourists trying to learn to swim in our beautiful lakes as adults. Seeing them struggle with what for us was such a simple task filled us with confusion and bemusement. This anecdotal introduction serves to highlight our lifelong fascination with intrinsic learning processes in general as well as on a detailed scale. These few experiences showed us, before we understood the significance, a certain propensity toward certain skills at certain ages. We began to learn that some developmentally dependent skills were easier to adopt than others and the way one relates to self-driven motivation. Some skills are imparted to us by teachers, mentors, and role models, like sports, ballet, or school subjects. Even so, there are also many things we seem to learn easier when left to figure it out on our own because we may be resistant to demonstrations. We may dislike theoretical explanations for relationships, or for learning to cook, even for some sports, which we prefer to learn by doing. Often children want to become independent from teachers and look for a self-chosen area to invest their own drive.

On one occasion Marguerite was invited to the slums of Cairo by a learned pediatric colleague Dr. U. Enayat. There, unexpectedly, she experienced one of the most challenging insights of her professional training. The outcast population of El Mokattam handled the sanitary needs of the 12 million inhabitant city by mapping the huge city into defined sectors to allow each family to take care of certain streets and bring the garbage back to the outskirts of the city before sunrise, there organizing the waste into varied piles. The children were put in charge of filling different boxes prepared for recycling of certain goods, thus supporting the family income.

© The Author(s), under exclusive license to Springer Nature
Switzerland AG 2022
M. Dunitz-Scheer, P. J. Scheer, *Child-led Tube-management and Tube-weaning*,
https://doi.org/10.1007/978-3-031-09090-5_1

The men and older boys would collect the garbage, the woman would sustain the household, and the children were expected to earn their keep. The outcast society had numerous children living in the muddy streets. Most women had given birth to 6–8 children before the age of 20! Marguerite had observed that breastfeeding ceased when infants learnt to walk; feeding the child after this was then taken over by the daughters of any given family. Bottle-feeding was non-existent, and mothers were not involved in transitioning to semi-solids nor solids or to drinking from cups or even learning to chew. We realized that any child able to walk and move independently was obviously also capable of eating various foods and with all the necessary skills by the age of 1 year.

Learning to eat isn't as simple as teaching a child to open its mouth when a spoon approaches it. The nuances of an infant *wanting* to open its mouth when the spoon is offered, or to wish and try to take over the task on its own, are far more complex. Learning to eat can be simple and easy when it happens "naturally" and needs no tuition. But viewed from a pediatric perspective, it is a multi-faceted process which requires experience and skills honed over time. Not to mention the need for a sensitive approach by caregivers in an appropriate setting during a specific but individually variable time window of the child's development.

So that's what it's all about! Learning to eat is a simple but potentially complicated task. Learning will happen when the process "happens as if by itself" and outsizes obstacles, difficulties, and anxieties involved.

This book highlights the distinct issue of children placed on temporary enteral nutrition support, ENS, due to their complex medical conditions. Special attention is given to their heroic transition from enteral to oral nutrition including the termination of all tube feeds. We will also be discussing the variety of adverse effects of "artificial feeding" defined in medical nomenclature as enteral nutrition support (ENS) and enteral nutrition tube feeding (ENT), sometimes also "gavage feeding." One notably worrying development in children who need ENT during their treatment in a NICU (neonatal intensive care unit) is their propensity toward tube dependency. Prolonged tube feeding may also have an impact on the emotional, social, psychological qualities and even motor development of the infant. Additionally, it imposes stress onto the family and creates a social isolation, or even discrimination, due to and constant exclusion of the child from its peers and the family in everyday life.

Our theoretical approach is necessarily child-led. Understanding this in detail will be a huge support in the process of swift and easy transition to drinking and eating independently. We do think that nearly every child placed on temporary intended ENT can learn to eat as nature prepared them to.

By eating all animals ingest the world. We taste and we smell it. We know how a doorknob tastes simply because we have tried it in early childhood. We know how carpets smell because we had our mouth and nose within. We are open systems: we need the influx of air, calories, and fluid. It's the innate knowledge of all fauna to interact with the world this way. Even severely handicapped children or children suffering from an untreatable, serious disease are most likely able to eat or to learn when assisted in a respectful way.

Children suffering from dysphagia (the inability to swallow safely) require immense caution due to the vulnerability they suffer during any act of swallowing. They will need to be excluded from natural learning to eat and drink, but this should be communicated openly with the parents at a well-chosen time and place and by giving an insight into neurological reasons. The evaluation of dysphagia has to be seen with a critical eye, as some of the tests available may provide incorrect results, e.g., if child cries while an X-ray swallow test is made, or it cries when a fluoro-endoscopy is done by an ENT—this may show inconclusive results and should be re-evaluated in the near future.

If pediatricians detect hearing impairment too late, speech development can be irreversibly impaired. If they detect visual impairment (like evolving amblyopy) too late, important treatment options might get be delayed or even missed.

To a certain extent the same is true for eating, smelling, biting, liking, tasting, chewing, and swallowing. If a child gets stuck on ENT, it will feel satiated all the time and not seek any alternative replacement. Later, it will withdraw when food is offered; it may even become frightened. The fear for both the infant and its caregivers is that it will end up being tube dependent. We present one effective remedy against development as described: EAT—an Early Autonomy Training, which allows the child itself to lead the way toward enjoying natural oral eating. The child knows best; nobody is more informed, not the therapists nor the MDs nor the parents. Only the child feels and knows when and how it can and will learn to eat.

To understand the meaning of the "language of the infant" like Hugh Lofting's fictional figure: "Doctor Doolittle" understands animals should be one of the prerequisites for any attending physician in this field. The couple Jaroslav (1920–1996) and Mechthild Papousek (1940–) invented a name for this phenomenon in parents terming it "intuitive parenting." Jaroslav, whom we could call a friend, documented his research fellowship at the National Institute for Mental Health in Bethesda, MA, USA, where he specifically looked at the vocal emissions, the tone, melody, and the vibrations of newborns voices. He could teach parents how to decipher the meaning of the acoustic cues of an infant merely 6 weeks old. This allowed parents to learn quickly, becoming mature and more capable for their next offspring. Babies have an ability to transmit at least four different vocal cues, asking for food, nurturing, comfort, or indicating unease or even pain. For pediatricians the ability to decipher the wishes and needs of a baby should be as good as it is in their parents. The features of an outpatient clinic can trigger immense anxiety for unprepared newborn. Then the infant cries uncontrollably, this making a discernible communication impossible. This, just as an example, is precisely why we weigh children attending our special treatment program in our day clinic in Graz fully clothed every second day, thus desensitizing them to the overwhelming unfamiliarity of the medical scene.

In the life of a child demanding early intensive medical care, a lot is done in order to save a child's life. These procedures, such as intubation, changing drips, and taking blood to test, are necessary but nevertheless frightening experiences for the young child. Flashbacks, a symptom of post-traumatic stress disorder (PTSD), may occur later, which are released (as we know from adults) already by odors or a specific light color or an image. In order to "understand" a proverbial baby, one must try to provide an encounter, which doesn't awaken these thoughts, thus leading to an agitation of the baby, and consequently in the parents making communication impossible.

We invite you to understand our approach, to observe and enjoy the way every child and its family find their own way out of tube dependency. This is our way of sharing our scientifically evaluated methods and portraying how we resolve family's distress. The topic of ENT is a budding and humble niche within modern pediatrics and involves medical, nutritional, social, and developmental issues. The topic is gaining increasing attention as more and more very-low-birthweight (VLBW) premature-born children survive and sometimes develop into medically fragile but stable infants. ENS is also becoming increasingly important in the care of medically fragile elderly people.

Another goal of this book is to bring awareness toward the complexity of any direct and indirect tube-related issues in patients, which can basically be of purely nutritional or entirely non-nutritive origin. The term "enterally fed" is confusing because it refers officially to any supplementary nutrition given by tube *or* taken by mouth. It needs to be explicitly known that this book is not addressing the issues of "oral supplementation," but has chosen to apply the term exclusively for bypassing food and fluids directly into the stomach or jejunum and use the term "tube-fed" synonymously to "enteral feeding." The subject matter we deal with is mainly infants and young children placed on temporary ENT whose medical conditions caused their lives to start in an intensive care unit (NICU and PICU) supported by high-tech machinery and pharmacology.

Most of these children would not be alive at all without the benefits of modern ENT: it is for this reason alone that our field is a necessity of all highly developed healthcare systems. The main causes for children receiving ENT are extreme prematurity, congenital anomalies requiring surgery, and genetic disorders. One of the most impacted groups we treat are infants born with a diaphragmatic hernia. Only by the invention of extracorporeal ventilation (ECMO), as extracorporeal renal support, it has become possible for those children to survive. With the support of this, they can undergo surgery as soon as the oxygenation of the blood is installed and are from then on unable to eat—consequently receiving ENT. Surprisingly most of these children show a very good outcome since they don't suffer from any additional brain injuries. To allow a child to lead a "normal" life, all medical support (like oxygen supplementation and ENS) must be stopped. This can of course only happen when the organ functions have recovered sufficiently. In nearly all cases, we successfully helped families because we were aware that the tube dependency was a reactive result of an inability to learn to eat during the natural phase of development. In most cases the feeding tubes are applied to newborns only for a short period of time like a few days or a few weeks. A permanent tube is only needed for rare diseases or children with progressive or irreversible neurological diseases or impairments or severe metabolic disorders and lastly for palliative treatment.

The main populations discussed in this book were once critically ill and now MFC who have stabilized and are able to live at home. They received a temporary tube with clear nutritional goals for a short period of time but became "stuck" on it and ended up being unintentionally long-term tube-fed. At this stage tube dependency develops; oral aversion and delayed eating development become significant issues as well. Normally parents are then transferred to SLPs, dieticians, and psychologists. In many of these cases, their support and advice is sufficient in helping the infant. We observe that pediatricians in the aftercare of a NICU treatment feel ill-equipped as they don't see nutrition as their primary field of interest. In such cases, the termination of ENS falls into the hands of professionals related to medical practice, which in cases of tube dependency may be insufficient. When suggestions and therapy don't lead to sufficient oral eating, families will look for more specialized help; that's where we come in. The externalities of tube feeding as well as some medical, technical, and nutritional considerations on the subject will be discussed in the first few chapters of this book. In the latter half, we will focus on the diversity of tube-related subjects like tube maintenance and management and finally tube weaning, which is the field of expertise we have contributed to.

The stimulation of the mouth, also termed oral rehabilitation as a starting point for the process of tube weaning, will be discussed later. One of our former PhD students Hannes Beckenbach [1] investigated the progress in non-mouth-related developmental tasks in 2010 "four categories of social competence: interactional and emotional development, self-help skills and social cognition." For his research he tested 51 children in the age range from 6 to 37 who were undergoing tube weaning 2 months before, at the end of a 3-week inpatient program and again 90 days after their first testing. Interestingly, all children improved in these categories after learning to sustain themselves exclusively orally. So general development was related positively to the normalization of oral intake. Intelligence was not a differentiating factor, indicating that socially transmitted impairments were improved, whereas inborn abilities or lack of them were not influenced by the transition to independent feeding.

Early childhood education venues often refuse children on ENT, due to the nursery teachers having neither the education nor the permission to feed a child using a tube. The daily tube feeding routine becomes disturbed by the needs of the children who don't take part in mealtimes and tend to refrain from collective sleeping after lunch. Food-related issues pose the risk of social isolation, not only the child but also its family. For the child, interactions in kindergarten have paramount meaning. It learns how to behave with peers, and how to play, finding its own place in society. Educating a child without kindergarten may lead to developmental issues in language and behavior, leading to distinct and basically avoidable discrimination of social skills.

We have heard countless stories of exasperated and desperate parents who feel alienated in public. Strangers may ask innocently what your child's problem is, simply because they are curious. Or they may give advice without being asked, like how they would feed that child, how they fed their own child, and how they think one should overcome feeding problems or make "political remarks" regarding how time changed and how children became more demanding and how they had been educated in times when food was sparse and imminent hunger was a daily threat. Most parents have heard these tropes hundreds of times and are simply sick of it, but helpless, exposed to unwanted and irrelevant advices. As a result, families tend to avoid what they enjoy most isolating themselves at home. Even finding a babysitter can be a big challenge as young students and people alike feel insecure handling a medical device.

We show later on that long-term tube-fed children suffer from adverse effects in more than 50% of all cases like retching and gagging and vomiting. Children with a PEG tube also experienced local granulation tissue or skin irritation [2]. An untrained babysitter would be unable to handle the liability; inevitably it is the parents who need pediatric nurses for nanny services when they want to have an evening out. Very few countries, like Germany or Switzerland, offer such services to parents of tube-fed children without costs beyond the average financial abilities. This becomes another source of social isolation of the affected families, isolated with their child.

This book is *not* judging. We discuss individual children (called in medical articles: "cases") and motivations and timings of why and when a feeding tube was placed. We don't want to get into the subject if tubes are seen as being necessary or not or "bad" and "invasive"; on the contrary, they can be very useful and a good medical intervention. We don't feel that we should take a stand in the very discussion, a discussion in which ideologies and beliefs are confronted with scientific medicine, which conclusively claims that without medical progress most of the children receiving ENT wouldn't be alive.

These discussions should be performed within an academic environment and are part of greater ideological conflicts. Normally they end when one's child is in desperate need of intensive care (ICU). Even so we are also aware of what some therapists within academic institutions claim. For one, the "nil by mouth," which uses as substance an assumption called "silent aspiration." This "silent aspiration" is unseen by definition and may lead to ongoing tube feeding and tube dependence. We ourselves had the most controversial discussions with pediatric colleagues all over the world and are grateful for every colleague who contributes to these discussions. We sometimes become advocates for the affected children, be it in a discussion with parents or out of mistrusting the local institutions or even between institutions and parents. If all parties try to support the MFCs as best as they can, we try to be as respectful as possible in all but one point: temporarily intended tubes must be taken out ASAP. We demand that even a plan for the end of ENT must be made in advance when the tube is inserted. On the premise that in an orthopedic operation a nail or another foreign body is inserted: on the day of the insertion, a day when the implanted device is taken out is established.

We lament at the lack of adequate help and support services for children showing obvious signs of tube dependency in most countries of the world. Our efforts try to combat it at every opportunity, be it by teaching or training or lecturing. This book was written in order to improve the understanding and treatment and justify effort for more tube maintenance and tube management services in high-tech health systems. Fortunately, this has led to increasing awareness for our subject and to the integration of terms like "tube dependence" and some of our methods like the invention "play picnic" in some children's hospitals.

We are certain that ENT has become an integrated part of medical care of its own right and that its indication and its positive nutritional effects outweigh accompanying unintended adverse effects. Unfortunately, side effects may worsen to such a degree that the intention of nutritional support goes wrong. This is the moment when the transition to oral intake and removal of the tube and ENT becomes an urgent necessity. The obstacle being that a feeding team may expect that a child compensates with a reduced ENS by oral intake right away. This leads to extensive in- or outpatient treatment and possibly even an inability to treat tube dependency. The time a child needs to compensate for its oral intake is challenging for all. For one the parents are afraid of weight loss especially in MFC children, therapists are sometimes not placed in charge of the child's weight, and MDs tend to refrain from the task of tube weaning. A slight weight loss may happen, but if a pediatrician supervises the weaning process, daily problems like dehydration and weight loss can be addressed and solved when necessary.

This book is dedicated to the children and their families that we met on our professional journey in the past four decades. We are happy that we met at exactly this stage in their lives.

The complexity of ENS/ENT is quite a new field for many professionals. We hope that our expertise and understanding will encourage many colleagues with an interest for this new field. Awarness for all needs of the children aside weight- and growth charts, an individually tailored feeding and weaning plan may lead to children, who will profit and not suffer unnecessarily often with the best intentions of feeding clinics and grow into a situation in which competence, confidence and knowledge outweighs anxiety and beliefs.

References

1. Beckenbach H. Developmental impact of a standardized tube weaning program (EAT, Early Autonomy Training; Graz Model for weaning tube dependency in infancy). Doctoral thesis, Medical Science, [online]. 2011. https://online.medunigraz.at/mug_online/wbAbs.showThesis?pThesisNr=30986&pOrgNr=14048, seen on 6 Jan 2022.
2. Pahsini K, Marinschek S, Khan Z, Dunitz-Scheer M, Scheer PJ. Unintended adverse effects of enteral nutrition support: parental perspective. J Pediatr Gastroenterol Nutr. 2016;62(1):169–73.

Assessment not only consists of reading but, just as importantly, observing as well. In our telemedical assessment, we ask parents to submit three 1-min videos of the child and its interactions with a parent. We ask for a feeding and a drinking attempt and a play situation. The length of the videos should not be more than a minute. It's incredible the amount that we can see from such a short clip. You see the environment in which the child lives, the kitchen where his meals are prepared, and whether the child is fed independently or takes part in a family meal. Furthermore, we see the in-/ability of the parents to feed their child. We recall a parent-child interaction in which the child showed no hunger but nevertheless was offered food on a spoon and turned its face away. Knowing that they were on video, the parents became forceful and pushed the spoon in the child's mouth. Looking at that video we knew that either the pressure to show how their child eats made this scene up or that the parents can't detect hunger and satiety cues in their child. Obstacles can be of psychological or so-called somatic nature. We recall a child, everything they ate or drank came out of its nose instantly after being fed.

The child drank happily but the milk came out of its nose after half a minute. We thought that it may be due to an esophageal obstruction or some other obstacle, which could be identified by X-ray. Pediatric surgeons investigated the results of the test and had to operate an esophageal stricture. A live or a recorded observation (which is often even better due to the family being in their home environment) is a prerequisite of every pre-assessment. The identification of an obstacle may not be so easy. We recall a child who was operated upon, due to being born without a part of the esophagus. The fistula between the esophagus and the trachea, which is a frequent finding in this enteral malformation, had been reportedly found and closed. When we began to feed that child, we observed that the infant would cough after a few sips regularly. We assumed that another undetected fistula may have been present. This happens often as the fistula starts as a very small hole, which can be overlooked even in an endoscopy. Re-evaluating was necessary; using a contrast fluid on water basis allowed the fistula to be detected and closed afterward. Why are we

© The Author(s), under exclusive license to Springer Nature Switzerland AG 2022
M. Dunitz-Scheer, P. J. Scheer, *Child-led Tube-management and Tube-weaning*,
https://doi.org/10.1007/978-3-031-09090-5_2

highlighting this case, because we strongly advocate that no feeding team can assume that every obstacle has been uncovered and addressed before they start. To get the permission to transition a child from ENS to oral feeding doesn't preclude any somatic obstacle from still being present; neither should one feel safe regarding psychological obstacles within parents or children. Insufficient development of the relationship with the child and intuitive parenting, according to the concept of the cited Papouseks, may pose even further difficulties.

During the treatment of any child, constant vigilance is necessary. One must be as aware as a commercial pilot. The concept of flight safety maintains one main tenant, every observation no matter where from is worth evaluating. In a study analyzing plane crashes, researchers often found in audio records that there was some sort of hint or observation, which could have saved the craft. After the crash it was too late to repair, undo, or salvage anything in order to commiserate catastrophe. It should be self-evident to require when treating a child, the same attention to detail and scrutiny as a flight team.

2.1   A Child's Underlying Medical History and Diagnosis Are Important But Not Always Relevant

As mentioned above the weaning team should know current diagnoses as well as all medical history since most children on ENS are so-called medically fragile children (MFC). The reason why we often term medical history as "not relevant" is to indicate that for whatever reason hooking a child onto the tube, the transition should be made when a temporarily indicated ENS has no somatic cause anymore. A 5-year-old boy who came to us from England, supported by a soccer team whose members were MDs and advocates, was diagnosed with "no brain." He suffered from a developmental disorder in his brain, blindness (amaurosis), and the inability to walk. He would sit in his pram making a revolving movement with his hands and shake his hand involuntarily. It wasn't known whether he could smell or taste. Numerous attempts to induce eating had been made. We reduced the amount of tube feedings (in our own way: quickly so that the child doesn't adjust to a hunger regime losing appetite) and offered him a variety of snacks. Leo began licking commercial potato chips. He didn't eat the chip itself; he merely relished the salt with the fat. In the beginning he maintained this habit through roughly five packets a day and was covered all over in chips. The child from head to toe, as well as its pram, was full of the remnants. Eventually the potato part of the chips dissolved, while he was licking and that's how he started to eat. We remember a benefit soccer game with the team of the psychiatric department of our Graz' University Hospital. Our support was required by the head of the department Prof. Dr. H.-P. Kapfhammer [1]; there one could see Leo, sitting at the corner full of chips being the star of the afternoon. Aftercare revealed that he learned to sustain himself orally, which may have added greatly to his quality of life.

Using this example, we advocate to give the child the wheel of its transition process. The child leads the way during transition; it chooses the nutrients from their quality, texture, and taste. Eating does not necessarily require one to utilize "intelligence"; even worms know how to eat. The brain is not needed to eat, nor is understanding why, or how, and what. Meaning knowledge on the content of a given food isn't necessary; eating comes by itself. The development of medicine gave MFCs a chance. Due to the lifesaving measures in early childhood and the pivotal impact of auxiliary ventilation, as well as the last 20 years of surfactant therapy, children survive who would have died before. This results in new challenges for physicians and paramedical personnel. Like in our example, the fear that Leo might aspirate or lose too much weight led to unsuccessful weaning attempts. It was necessary to believe in Leo and not interfere too much in his choices and find his own gentle way to learn how to eat. The anxiety that he may choke on a chip was unnecessary. The disgust experienced by others as seeing him covered in sloppy remnants of chips was a problem of the adults. Leo couldn't care less what people thought. As one doesn't typically find any amaurotic children learning to eat in literature, we were exploring new ground. Our path was chosen by Leo, and our strength was the confidence we had in him. Fear and assumptions regarding a child's ability to learn to eat shouldn't be our guides in this journey.

2.2   Respect the Genetically Determined Developmental Pathways

Medically fragile children like the forementioned Leo bear a variety of genetic abnormalities. After the detection and complete mapping of the gene, we know that every being has a couple of variations in his genome. One could say that nearly 98% of genomes are the same, and the other 2% all of us have deviations from a statistical norm. Most of these changes have no impact on the production of proteins as they are "silent"; somehow, they are backed up by genetic information or simply are not taking part in the system of synthesis of specific proteins, enzymes, and other biochemical processes in us. In some cases, researchers observe a clinical feature, which suggests a syndrome. Before the advance of genetic science, doctors observed a variation in posture, facial deformation, or a combination of defects and gave these changes a name, mostly the name of the first researcher who found this combination. Family trees disclosed whether the defects were hereditary or not. Today genetic assessments using various techniques detect more variations than clinical-morphologic studies. In tube-fed children, we have a large concentration of genetic syndromes, which we have to address individually. We find in literature that it's sometimes assumed that children suffer rare from syndromes. I can't learn to eat. Sometimes a researcher assumes that a child can't smell and due to that will never learn to eat. Sometimes, like in syndromes showing dwarfism, it is assumed that the child needs only a little food and has nearly no appetite. The problem with research is that genetic researchers are not so much interested in clinical features but rather genetic assessment. This may be why the newly arising clinical symptoms are not assessed, because one paper cites in this respect another one, and "less appetite" and "inability to eat" are transferred uncritically from one result to another. When we look at the child, its parents, and their actions, we need not know too much regarding genetic testing. Yes, we do see clinical features and sometimes detect a genetic disorder in the same way our ancestors did, by simply observing the child.

Even without discernible defects or syndromes, every child has its own genetically determined traits, which enables it to be quick or slow, witty or dull, etc. Some children could be seen as traumatized by the procedures they were submitted to in intensive care. Some have surprising predilections. Judy Mennella [2, 3] from Philadelphia, has shown that children being submitted to intensive care tend to prefer savory food. The reason is unknown, but it may be a result of what they smelled during the early phase of life. Sometimes the preterm birth is caused by genetic disorders; sometimes the ripeness of the given child is inhibited by genetic specificities. In all cases, the genetic situation is determined by the generations before them, by the genetic apparatus provided by its parents, and at the end by the expression of genes within the child itself. All these factors form a specific child with its own strengths and shortcomings. We tend to focus on the abilities, and we observe preferably what a child is able to do rather than his handicaps.

In conclusion, never believe what literature tells you about a specific syndrome. Never assume, respect the volatility of learning, stay vigilant, but never give up.

Eating needs a lot of abilities, take your time, and give the child its space and a fair chance to make some changes toward more normality.

References

1. Fuchshuber J, Hiebler-Ragger M, Kresse A, Kapfhammer HP, Unterrainer HF. The influence of attachment styles and personality organization on emotional functioning after childhood trauma. Front Psychiatry. 2019;5(10):643. https://doi.org/10.3389/fpsyt.2019.00643. PMID: 31543844; PMCID: PMC6739441.
2. Mennella JA, Bobowski NK. The sweetness and bitterness of childhood: insights from basic research on taste preferences. Physiol Behav. 2015;152(Pt B):502–7. https://doi.org/10.1016/j.physbeh.2015.05.015. Epub 2015 May 20. PMID: 26002822; PMCID: PMC4654709.
3. Mennella JA, Jagnow CP, Beauchamp GK. Prenatal and postnatal flavor learning by human infants. Pediatrics. 2001;107(6):E88. https://doi.org/10.1542/peds.107.6.e88.

Presentation of the EAT Concept

EAT (Early Autonomy Training) is a system we champion, which highlights the child's agency in the act, as eating is inherently—when not disturbed—a genetically programmed self-driven ability developed in social environments in which eating happens naturally. Any requirement for support, be it sensory, emotional, or functional, needs some sort of practice or training on the side of the child within a sensitive and suitable social context. Adults are involved but need to offer some reasonable space for the process. Infants need assistance in eating and drinking in their first years of life but mastering more mature and complex skills only works when they actively involve themselves. Unlike sleeping, breathing, or peeing, which is autonomous and instinctual, drinking and eating need to be actively "learnt." In children who grew up during month of their early life and are unable to drink, either due to prematurity or illness, an active step of motivation and decision needs to occur on the child's side.

This approach of looking at the issue of early eating disorders from mainly the child's perspective was introduced by us using the new term EAT. As we have already mentioned EAT stands for **E**arly **A**utonomy **T**raining. When trying to understand eating issues, caregivers and doctors alike tend to see and identify with the topic from an adult perspective. They decide on the choice and composition of the food offered, the number of calories, quality, texture, etc. Whether the child consents to the nutrition and its inherent goals, whether it wants to be the receiver, or whether it wishes to cooperate and eventually be grateful is not explicitly considered From the child's perspective, it's an internal communication with its stomach, the hunger-satiation centers in the brain, its general mood, as well as optical attractivity and smells and the social atmosphere at any given moment that will influence its motivation to eat or not. Terms used by adults such as "food refusal" and "oral aversion" suggest that something was offered and then somehow fails. The terminology isn't suggesting an active decision such as "I would prefer not," but rather as disorder, bad behavior, or a failure.

In an adult-adult relationship the situation would simply be one in which the receiver states: "I don't want your offer!" be it a TV set, some food, or anything else. It would be seen as a natural option in reaction to an offer, whereas in children it is seen and judged differently. The adult intention to know what's good for a child is hardly ever questioned. There is an incredible onus on the child to consent due to it being associated with its very survival. What we miss is that the child's refusal may be intelligent or well justified, perhaps the child knows something we don't, e.g., its gut may currently not be able to digest the food. Refusal can only happen if somebody offers something to another who doesn't want it. In a caregiver-child relationship, it's assumed that the parent may offer food or drink without it being requested and furthermore that the child's refusal shouldn't be taken seriously due to higher priorities such as obeying and abstract weight goals. Many professionals support this conviction and even impose stress on parents because a child "drops out of the line in which the child was born on the growth-chart." Thus, a logical and physiologically motivated reaction of a given child is interpreted as a "refusal" or "resistance." The child's own feelings of being over-fed to gain weight and make development possible is not taken seriously because adults decide for the child.

Unlike forementioned personnel, we like to assume that refusal of an offer of food is an intelligent, precisely targeted active and goal-oriented decision, which is a result of diverse intentions and feelings of the child including recognition of smell, texture, hunger, and satiety as well as a general reaction to the situation. In movies we often see romantic dinners spoiled due to a photo of a former lover being discovered or a specific dish evoking bad memories. Suddenly the romance is gone, and one finds an unsavory unrepairable situation. We think that the child has agency in its own consumption, not only they are fed, but they also take the food internally and either may be able to digest it or not. The individualized respect and the attempt to understand the child has been our backbone for assessment and treatment of early feeding disorders since the late 1980s and early 1990s.

At the time, literature on early feeding problems in earlier years were of a mainly psychiatric origin (focused on mother-child interaction as in the pioneering work by Irene Chatoor [1, 2] in infant psychiatry). These ideas didn't seem applicable for us dealing with the majority of medically fragile children referred to our University Hospital in Graz at the time. Infants, toddlers, and younger children suffered from various issues in insufficient oral intake, sometimes growth retardation and insufficient intake volumes. Most of our cases at the time came from the NICU after preterm birth or due to genetic malformations. Chatoor's children on the other hand were part of middle-class families around Washington, DC. Nowadays children are born to older parents than hundred years ago. Parents are involved in work, and in the case of the Washington, DC, outpatient clinic even careers. So, a disturbance or an inhibited development due to eating problems didn't fit into their timeframes. The children we took care of in Graz came from all social backgrounds, but the physical ailment is what made eating in the first place impossible. We recall a child suffering from a Pierre-Robin complex named Robert. He was treated within the NICU for 6 weeks, and treatment ended while the child still needed it's nasogastric feeding tube. The Department of Neonatology's aftercare clinic still found him tube dependent after 6 more months. Trying to introduce oral feeding failed (advice like "offer food on a spoon" or "skip one or two feedings—hunger is going to kick in" or "you must be patient—time will solve the problem" was given), so they sent him to our clinic.

Robert was afraid of food as were his parents. To soothe both parties, we thought to demonstrate how to feed Robert. Irene Chatoor taught us that it is devastating for parents when they witness a nurse or any professional feed their baby and succeed where they had failed for weeks with the best of intentions. Their self-esteem becomes even lower than it might have been already. So, we concentrated on the situation: reducing anxiety, which came on the parents' side from the fear that Robert might aspirate and suffer from a lung infection subsequently. On Robert's side, a baby bottle which was equipped with a Haberman feeder [3] (an especially designed feeder, which uses cleft and gum to receive milk from the bottle) was unknown. He associated most unknown things brought to his mouth as possibly causing pain. The child's intuitive reaction was turning away from the food. The head of the Department of Neonatology was a friend of the grandparents. He came to our ward daily to see how we proceeded. He saw that in our approach, Robert was in charge himself. Even being an only 8-month-old child, he decided himself when he wanted what.

After some days, it became clear that a baby bottle was impossible, the developmentally defined time window for bottle-feeding had closed already. We used a soft spoon, which was held by Robert and his caretaker. Most of the content would end up spilled on his clothes or mother's apron. We didn't allow any other devices, not even a bib. Every meal had both participants covered in stains, and clothes had to be changed afterward. Even the bedsheets were spoiled, which was a problem for the nurses. Robert led us all through a journey in reducing his anxiety. ENS was reduced accordingly, gently but swiftly, and hunger kicked in. Robert started to want to eat according to his own requests. One spoon offered too fast was as bad as if the spoon was too slow. After a week of reducing stress (some of which being our own due to the supervision of the head of the NICU), Robert had managed to eat and learned that not every object approaching his mouth will eventually be pushed forcefully into him. We must thank Robert for the lessons he taught us. We want to understand the meaning within the cues expressed by the child itself. The word "cues" is specially meant for nonverbal signals, which may even be expressed by a preverbal baby or by any person or even animal. The understanding of cues is learnt in everyday life quite automatically. Parents of a first baby need approximately 4–6 weeks to become adequate in interpreting the baby's expressions.

If these interpretations are interrupted or inaccurate, the interactions themself become equally disturbed. When a baby is born prematurely, it needs medical help; it may even be ventilated and put into an incubator within a NICU. In such a life-threatening situation, the expression of discernable signals is reduced to pain and discomfort. Heidi Als [4] found that the non-development of differentiated signals is also due to the medical surroundings in which the baby exists: constant light (in order to observe any change of vital signs), puncturing of the calf without the awareness of the baby, and machinery emitting a lot of sound. These factors could and have been adjusted according to Heidi's findings in most countries.

On the parent's side, the unusual environment of a neonatal intensive ward may lead to apprehension and insecurity possibly causing them to even distance themselves from their baby. When dismissal from the ward is imminent, a brief overview of subsequent steps is offered by the medical staff. Upon discharge, parents may be overwhelmed by the tasks that are required to master on their own now. The baby's signals may also not be properly developed, or it did not learn them yet. The emitting and the deciphering of cues is not developed and may become even further impacted. When a baby needs auxiliary oxygen or is put on ENS, the development of differentiated signals is even further inhibited. On the parent's side, the recognition of the subtle difference between signals may not work, and thus the baby will not develop corresponding tactics when not understood. A simpler example may be a developmentally stunted signal exchange when mothers suffer from a postpartum depression. In these cases, the understanding doesn't occur as mothers are unable to decipher the baby's signals. As they respond to every cry or frown with feeding or cuddling, the baby's signals don't develop diversely and appropriately. In the beginning of our own work, we observed intrusive and inappropriate feeding techniques be it by nurses or parents; this is how we learnt what was wrong. Neither of us are Austrian born: Marguerite was born in Bethesda, Massachusetts, in the USA and Ronny in Tel-Aviv, so local customs like patting a baby on its back and head during feeding in order to stimulate its sucking were unfamiliar to us.

The infant-led approach seemed obvious to us but was clearly contrasted to the mainstream literature prior to 2000. Papers were full of mother blaming[1] claiming that emotional instability such as postpartum depression, insensitivity, attachment issues, bonding inability, and various other problems on the mother's side inhibited the development of a natural intuition. Life-threatening levels of malnutrition and the inability to thrive in newborns were considered a direct consequence of the mother's nonsupportive behavior. The "state of the art" treatment was therefore, and unfortunately often still is in many places, the recommendation for mothers to seek psychological or even psychiatric help. In our research we found that this so-called psychiatric disorder fads away when the child started eating [5]. The eating problem in itself was the cause of the psychic disturbance, creating a sort of "chicken-and-egg" problem. Did the expression of discomfort or insecurity from the mother cause the baby's food refusal or did the food refusal in turn cause the mother's emotional issues. We argue that only the inability to feed one's baby on the mother's side would be caused by psychiatric illness. In our study, we could show that mothers became healthy again when feeding worked. In some institutions, mothers were even separated from their children because it was assumed that the mother-baby

---

[1] "Whereas Pollitt et al. (1975) found that overt pathology was not more likely in FTT mothers than in mothers of normally thriving infants, most authors support the presence of psychosocial problems in FTT mothers (Fraiberg 1975; Evans 1972; Drotar et al. 1979)." From: New Directions in Failure to Thrive: Implications for Research and Practice (pp. 235–258). A Developmental Classification of Feeding Disorders Associated with Failure to Thrive: Diagnosis and Treatment.

interaction itself was causing food refusal. Sometimes this may have aided mothers in their personal turmoil, but rarely did this have a positive effect on feeding issues. Often it resulted in more permanent separation, even resulting in the child being placed in a foster home. The reestablishment of a working mother-child relationship requires a functioning signal exchange system, thus making it extremely sensitive to the disturbances of the NICU, the hospital, and afterward. To support its development, an understanding of the baby's cues is a necessary hurdle for parents to be able to truly comprehend their baby. When inaccurate or insincere communication becomes regular, it may very well result in a disorder.

From the early 1980s to the end of 2010, we were employed by the large and prestigious University Hospital for Children and Adolescents in Graz, Austria. The hospital serves as a first-line children's hospital as well as a third-line university center for more specific diseases, which are also a subject of the hospital's research. The hospital serves a catchment area of approx. two million people and is meant to be the final salvation for those seeking a cure. We saw patients at risk of life-threatening weight loss; we witnessed parents feeling trapped and helpless because their child would neither eat nor accept ENS. Being pediatricians, we look at the child first. From a medical perspective, it is the child itself who needs support, not only the parents. We quickly realized the interaction between the feeding person and receiving child was somehow uneven, likely the result of a distorted interaction. The thoughts and emotions of the caretaker were motivated by medical and paramedical notions; the child felt instincts, which were mostly those concerned with satiation. Caretakers after being instructed to change their behavior become more insecure than before. Sometimes an aspect of feeding is altered, be it the child's formula, the bottle, and/or the seating position of the mother or the child's posture. Trial and error is a feasible approach to managing a feeding problem. Nevertheless, we assume that every therapist, be it a MD or a SLP or a physiotherapist, has to observe before giving any advice. Ideas from textbooks and training courses may be a good basis for therapeutic practice, but observation and empathy are needed if mistakes are to be avoided. Parents and their children were caught in the turmoil of contradictory advice, adding to their existing sense of insecurity. Parents imposed pressure on their children during feeding, leading to a great deal of stress for the child. Parents got endless advice on the seemingly "simple issue of food." Every staff member felt competent to impart advice resulting in even further confusion.

Pediatricians use to refer these families to psychologists who aren't typically trained in nutrition as this is true for a couple of paramedics like physiotherapists and even speech language therapists (SLT). Even dieticians may have no training in recognition, and therapy of interactional family dynamics and nutritionists may focus mainly on the intake protocol and not on the behavioral aspects of food refusal. Both paramedics may have no knowledge of fine-tuning of nutrition but are nevertheless expected to give suitable advice to insecure parents. Sometimes dieticians were not involved in planning nutrition at all. The modification of nutritional plans rested with the MDs—resulting in a therapeutic approach of the paramedics where the cornerstone of tube weaning could not be touched. Only when dieticians or SLTs were in charge to change the intake plan, their work could succeed. In most cases advice ended when it came to ENT reduction or when resistance to oral intake were dominant. Only the presence of medical and psychological competence makes successful therapy of tube dependency possible.

It was the recognition of this illogical situation that brought about our own method of observing the infant itself and focusing on nothing but its cues and reactions to tiny changes; it seemed the only way forward to help the family out of this trap.

We were following a pediatric developmentally focused psychodynamic approach in contrast to behaviorally oriented psychotherapy, which was at the beginning of the century advocated by Benoit and her most cited study from Toronto [6]. While we were experimenting with this seemingly revolutionary approach, we realized that the observation and analysis of feeding situations could be influenced by sharing our findings with the family including the child, who understood not the psychodynamic content but the emotions in the room. As much as possible, we tried to interpret nothing. Sentences like "this may be the result of your…" or "the cause may lie in your own childhood …" or even "perhaps it's not that simple after all that you have endured during pregnancy and labor …" were avoided completely. When reflecting the interactional process during eating with the family, we could see small but continuous changes with positive effects related to drinking and eating. The best Diane Benoit did was to highlight the problem for the medical world. Her manual-driven therapeutic process, which was offered by instructed students during half a year, was a very good first try. We tried to improve her therapy even using her statistical analysis method for publishing our first cohort of patients [7] and after having visited the institution in which she developed her therapy (Toronto's children's hospital). During meals we were present ourselves, not because we had too much spare time, but had nearly no personnel when we started. In contrast to the expected way of pediatricians, we felt the need to step back (if the child was in a stable condition) and *observe* the nature of the feeding problem. Observing means a nonintrusive, sensitive, tuned in behavior omitting any judgment. Thus, we gained a bountiful source of new and useful information. We could, as MDs, evaluate the quantity and quality of nutrition as well as the state of the child and its growth over time, holding back on interventions like putting the child into stressful examinations or even oral intrusions.

The traditional form of a hospital assessment would have been stripping the child, performing a complete bodily examination, weighing, measuring of height and head circumference, taking a blood array, prescribing X-ray swallow test, and additionally a fluoroscopy and—if any results point to a severe malfunction—additional intrusive tests like gastroscopy. It's understood that we did all of that if any hint showed the necessity for them. Bodily exams were made in all cases only after a trustworthy relationship could be established. Most children came to us after they had undergone all these tests—in some cases, we detected pathophysiological problems, for example, when a child vomited always during mouth and nose after eating happily (we found a ligament of Treitz, which made propulsion of the food at a certain point impossible). If the results were without pathological findings or inconclusive like most X-ray swallow tests and fluoroscopy, as the child may have stirred during it, or the test was terminated due to non-cooperativity, observation of the eating situation could help sometimes more. Seeing refusal, retching, or signs of a dumping disorder or inadequate offers by parents or simply understanding that a situation is too stressful for eating gave us the opportunity to interact with parents sometimes without adding stress by applying medical tests.

It is useful to support the child by providing a secure environment and offer confidence to both the parents and the child. The child itself will make its next step toward orality whenever it is ready. The institutional pressure during our observational approach toward a non-eating child, demanding parents and colleagues who looked mainly at weight charts, was simply immense. The expectation to do something effective immediately was strong, making it nearly impossible to give a child a fighting chance itself to get out of artificial tube feeding, which at this point had sustained the child for months or years. The assumption that sufficient feeding leads to a better intellectual development and even to healthier weight and height is typical in pediatrics, but it's only true of hunger [8]. The understanding of unexpected adverse effects of ENS is sparse since the number of patients on ENS of each doctor and hospital are small. Khan et al. [9] published a study showing that one-third of all patients exclusively tube-fed for most of their life were suffering from moderate to severe malnutrition. It is especially relevant in these cases that the idea of discontinuation of the winning horse, i.e., the tube, needs to be re-evaluated [10].

Let us outline and summarize some cornerstones of the EAT concept:

(a) No diagnostic assumptions before meeting the child (the medical history and narrative of parents about their perception of the presenting problem is not necessarily the problem of the child) itself.
(b) Don't try to meet the parent's unrealistic expectations as top priority; the adult mindset and its possible transition might need more support than the child's oral skills.
(c) No therapeutic actions before a thorough analysis of the history and the current state.
(d) Try to understand what has been preventing eating development to unfold naturally up to now from both the child's, the parent's, and the responsible medical and therapeutic teams' perspective.

We strongly advocate gathering all information available on the child. This process starts at pregnancy followed by delivery and even through the postpartum period. Findings are collated regarding inborn errors of metabolism as well as genetic disturbances, and finally reports of therapists are produced. To make it complete, we developed a questionnaire at the university before Notube started including at first the address of the home-based pediatrician. This is an indication that cooperation is important, and only when we decide against the ideas of the local doctor to wean a child, then we know that the cooperation might be impossible. The questionnaire consists of three parts: pre- and post-natal history, facts regarding ENS and its possible side effects, and volume of food, how it's given, and whether it had a positive or a detrimental effect on the child. The psychological and social part asks about age, illnesses, and reactions toward ENS of the parents. This allows us to get an overview of the child and its family. Parents need approximately 10–20 min to answer the questionnaire, so we get an invaluable impression in a short time. Contradictory or misleading assumptions for tube weaning may be cleared up after receiving the questionnaire avoiding situations where the child is able to eat and drink sufficiently but is kept on ENS because of anxiety to wean by parents or medical teams. We refuse any attempt to change the food intake of a given child without this crucial information.

This seems to be a natural and logical approach, and everyone would say so. Why do we stress this point so thoroughly? Because we visited dozens of institutions around the world which treated children, and unaware of the anamnesis, they wanted to subject it to transition. In one case a genetic defect wasn't discovered due to the morphological signs suggesting a variant of facial composition and expression. These things can happen, and whoever claims it doesn't is probably lying. But we saw children where the defect was known, by the attending pediatrician, and not by the members of the weaning team, sometimes because in the team there was no MD. Therefore, we employ a pre-weaning assessment, performed by one or two members of our pediatric team of four, and one of our extremely knowledgeable clinical psychologists (Dr. Sabine Marinschek and Dr. Karoline Pahsini both MAs in natural sciences and PhDs in medical sciences) is requested to evaluate all the information given by parents online and reject the assessment process if information is inconclusive or incomplete. Since our clients have come from 53 different countries up until now, language is a pivotal issue. Our staff is proficient in German, English, French, and Spanish. If a letter from a hospital, let's say from Prague, is in Czech, we ask for translation or at least a summary made by the parents into one of our four languages. We strongly advise all involved to assume that one has understood the important features of a letter in a language unknown to him or her. This may result in a misunderstanding and may subsequently endanger the child.

All information should be read with as much care as possible. When starting the transition process, one should summarize the information received and ask for consent of parents. If a child is old enough to understand, and the therapist is reluctant to discuss these matters in presence of the child because it might be ashamed or have difficult recollections, then a meeting with parents alone should be made to exchange existing knowledge and eventually complete the anamnesis. We can recall several instances where it was necessary to get in touch with the pediatrician in the hometown of the child to get further information. In Haifa, Israel, we met, for example, a child who could cope with eating, especially sweet and crunchy things, but was unable to swallow liquids. Additionally, the child suffered from a rare kind of diabetes. This was why the mother gave him every half an hour some water with cornstarch using his PEG. When discussing this "diagnosis" or more accurately this belief, we were told that the finding had been discovered by an X-ray swallow test. The physicians were unable to find the actual test on their desk or computer. We decided to give the child a drink, and surprisingly he drank from a sport bottle, which we had in our hand, and subsequently was able to be weaned easily.

To conclude, certainly some assumptions of attending pediatricians or paramedical staff can and should sometimes be overruled to achieve the aim of a child eating.

This should only be done when being fully aware of all the findings and conclusions of the MDs and other persons who had met and treated the child before its referral to you.

References

1. Chatoor I, Egan J. Nonorganic failure-to-thrive and dwarfism due to food refusal: a separation disorder. J Am Acad Child Psychiatry. 1983;22:294–301.
2. Chatoor I. Infantile anorexia nervosa: a developmental disorder of separation and individuation. J Am Acad Psychoanal. 1989;17:43–64.
3. Campbell AN, Tremouth MJ. New feeder for infants with cleft palate. Arch Dis Child. 1987;62(12):1292. https://doi.org/10.1136/adc.62.12.1292. PMID: 3435170; PMCID: PMC1778644.
4. Als H. Developmental care in the newborn intensive care unit. Curr Opin Pediatr. 1998;10(2):138–42. https://doi.org/10.1097/00008480-199804000-00004. PMID: 9608890.
5. Dunitz M, Scheer PJ, Kvas E, Macari S. Psychiatric diagnosis in infancy: a comparison. Infant Ment Health J. 1996;17:12–24.
6. Benoit D, Madigan S, Lecce S, Shea B, Goldberg S. Atypical maternal behavior toward feeding-disordered infants before and after intervention. Infant Ment Health J. 2001;22:611–26. https://doi.org/10.1002/imhj.10221.
7. Trabi T, Dunitz-Scheer M, Kratky E, Beckenbach H, Scheer PJ. Inpatient tube weaning in children with long-term feeding tube dependency: a retrospective analysis. Infant Ment Health J. 2010;31(6):664–81. https://doi.org/10.1002/imhj.20277. PMID: 28543064.
8. https://www.feedingamerica.org/hunger-blog/3-ways-hunger-affects-your-body, seen on 02/13/2021.
9. Khan Z, Marinschek S, Pahsini K, Scheer P, Morris N, Urlesberger B, et al. Nutritional/growth status in a large cohort of medically fragile children receiving long-term enteral nutrition support. J Pediatr Gastroenterol Nutr. 2016;62(1):157–60.
10. Marinschek S, Pahsini K, Scheer PJ, Dunitz-Scheer M. Long-term outcomes of an interdisciplinary tube weaning program: a quantitative study. J Pediatr Gastroenterol Nutr. 2019;68(4):591–4.

Focus on the Child and Don't Get Distracted by Additional Information Offered for Free or on Demand!

4

It may be helpful to know whether the child on ENS was observed by ultrasound in the womb as HF Prechtl and his successors have shown us [1]. Additional signs of a well-functioning neurological swallow coordination during pregnancy can be observed when the fetus deals of its amniotic fluid. In cases with an excess of amniotic fluid, a preterm caesarean might become necessary. Observing the swallowing in unborn children proves that they can drink. When additionally able to breath sufficiently after delivery, a newly born infant moves swiftly to the mother's breast. When turning its head from side to side, the mother's nipple is stimulated and milk flow is induced. This movement is called rooting and exists instinctually in all mammals. It may be interpreted as a hunger cue or at least as an inborn drive for attachment. When the mother-child cuddling after birth is impossible due to physical issues including the child's need for an incubator or even auxiliary ventilation, hunger cues can't be emitted. Sometimes the cues are very subtle, and at times endotracheal ventilation needs to put the child into "sleep" to withhold its resistance against mechanical ventilation, thus possibly enhancing the risk of brain hemorrhage. In such and similar situations, the child receives sufficient nutrition by a venous drip and/or ENS and is never hungry. There can be exceptions where placental insufficiency brought insufficient nutritional support to the child. Therefore, mechanically ventilated children don't learn to discriminate hunger from unease or even pain. Researchers [2] have contributed to that observation with the concept of allodynia. This means that infants (as well as elderly people) cannot always detect the exact origin of their own discomfort. They feel a pain in an unidentifiable place, and this feeling will thus include their whole being. They cry but are not able to express why. This is true for the discomfort of hunger as well; babies often emit a sound, which simply cannot be interpreted correctly. Even in healthy children, the sound of a baby crying without a sufficient answer from caregivers tends to become uniform. One can observe that in an airplane when parents can't get off and can't help their baby with their pain caused by under pressure in the middle ear, babies will signal that they are in pain. After a few minutes, this sound changes to a uniform cry, which

M. Dunitz-Scheer, P. J. Scheer, *Child-led Tube-management and Tube-weaning*,
https://doi.org/10.1007/978-3-031-09090-5_4

doesn't indicate ear pain anymore but becomes like a basso-sostenuto in the opera—unspecific and uniform. At this point we hear soothing remarks from the mother carrying her baby in the aisle, like "after landing everything will be okay" or "it won't be long now" which are inevitably futile. Allodynia has taken over the baby's whole existence. The reason for this explanation is to highlight that we know that the development of hunger cues may take time on the babies' side as well as the recognition of their very subtle signs by parents. To detect these soft signs parents, need support.

We wonder whether SLTs who work in and around the oral cavity in order to stimulate eating and reduce oral resistance against an offered bottle or spoon are helpful. Our approach differs. We think that observing minor cues of hunger (as after reducing tube feeds swiftly) may be more helpful. If a child is hungry and in a safe environment, it can begin learning. If at first the uncomfortable feeling of hunger can't be detected correctly, professionals and parents should retreat. To cuddle one's child reduces insecurity and anxiety but doesn't help the child to learn that this unspecific discomfort is in fact hunger. Food must be offered in an age-appropriate way without any kind of force, harassment, or intention of living up to the parents' expectations. It is the sole and exclusive task of the infant to establish a connection between its adverse feelings and its relief by ingesting food. Therapists and parents can support this process by eating themselves (which we explain in depth in the chapter: play picnic). Hearing a child after a lengthy stay on ENS emitting its first sound, which can be interpreted as a hunger cue, or listening to an infant who says for the first time "I am hungry" "I want an ice-cream", is incredibly rewarding. The path to this moment might be bumpy and long—but the moment is priceless.

4.1   Respect the Child's Own and Basic Drive for Autonomy

A child is a person of its own right. It is of crucial importance to respect the full meaning of this assumption. It might sound obvious but needs to be accepted and translated into every single interaction with and about and around the infant. The sentence "humans are all born as preterm" is true. Newborns, even born healthy at term, are in fact helplessly dependent, especially when it comes to nutrition and growth. When we focus on eating and drinking, the child itself plays the main role. It's them who know what, how, and how much he/she likes. It's the baby who must accept the food into its mouth, process it in the mouth, submit it to swallowing, and digest it. It's not the mother, nor the father, nor medical personnel who can do that for the baby. When medical issues are dominant, there are a couple of measures to bypass that: one can feed a baby using an intravenous drip. Research shows that this is possible only for short periods of time like a few days. If it is done for too long, liver problems and side effects may become so severe that they outweigh the intended benefits.

In such situations, the baby may get ENS administered by a nasogastric tube in the beginning, ending up perhaps with a PEG or even a JPEG. All the applied medical procedures have side effects, which make the oral intake of nutrition, if anatomically possible, the best way to feed a baby. Sometimes the expectations of adults don't fit the baby's abilities or feelings. This is well-known with healthy babies who are expected to transit to carrots or fruit purees at the age of 4–5 months. Mothers are told to offer their children variations of new food to supply them with all the necessary nutrients. Some babies don't want to eat from a spoon, others dislike the sour taste of fruits, and some even refrain from everything but their mother's milk—these are very common problems in any pediatric clinic.

In medically fragile patients, MFCs, their defense efforts might become even more pronounced. Maybe they just survived various medical interventions which were painful or at the very least uncomfortable. Perhaps the child needed auxiliary ventilation after being discharged, having to wear an oxygen device in its nose, which made smelling nearly impossible. Or perhaps the child was submitted to a particularly forceful feeding attempt to change from ENS to orality. The reasons why a given child reacts to food in a certain way can be numerous and hard to narrow down. Research [3] found that the eating-swallow coordination becomes dysfunctional after permanent tube feeding. The gag reflex can sometimes move to the front and may even start at the lips (normally it's situated in the rear of the mouth at the velum palatinum). One believes that even just touching the lips with food may already evoke a gagging reflex. The gagging reflex is a necessary feature of every living creature and hinders the aspiration of fluids and food into the lungs.

When food arrives at the velum palatinum, it is detected as unwelcome; gagging and spitting may save one's life. In children who haven't ever eaten, the gagging reflex may be triggered prematurely, so that every approaching food leads to this reaction. One can imagine this by remembering a situation with severe nausea, where even the smell of food could trigger gagging or even vomiting. The same is true for children who, for whatever reason, are unable to eat. To overcome these complex and aversive feelings and reactions, some children need a lot of time. The child's pace may seem to be too slow for parents and the feeding team. It is crucial to respect the time a child needs to get acquainted with the smell, touch, and textures of new food. If the child feels nausea at the sight of food, one should not push. During the play picnic (which will be described in a later chapter) offered at our Eating-School (which will also be closely described in an own chapter), we are content when a child starts by merely observing. It may be the case, as Petr, a Czech 5-year-old boy, showed us that he at first needed to leave the room after a few minutes. We could change that by influencing his loving father. Whenever food was offered, the very slim man in his 40s used to leave the room where the buffet was displayed, went outside, and smoked a cigarette. We asked the father to smoke after the meal or refrain from smoking while attending the ES, changing the garden of the school to a non-smoker area. As Petr witnessed his father eating in the given room, he stayed with him. The smell of food dominated the child's senses even when being close to his father, before then he only smelled smoke when he cuddled him. This was a new experience for the father, his son, and for us. Father and son both had to overcome their food resistance and accomplished the task together.

4.2   Use a Multidimensional Perspective (Physical, Functional, and Psychological)

It's never one single cause, which makes eating impossible. There are different reasons why a child doesn't/will not/can't eat. That is why the team dealing with a child should consist of more than one profession. Pediatricians will address the intrauterine life, the neonatal period, the current medical status, and problems with breathing and defecation which might in itself give the child a constant feeling of nausea or at least saturation. The volume, type, and caloric content of food are also a pediatric concern. Together with a dietician, the composition of food will be discussed. Especially for a transition process from ENS to orality questions like "sufficient nutrients" or hydration arise and need to be answered. A physiotherapist may investigate the child's posture during meals. Reclining positions may be adequate during breastfeeding, but a child eating by itself needs to have an upright position. It's recommended that the feeding person sees the child's mouth while offering food. Some parents learned to keep the child very close to them, sometimes even holding in such a way that it hinders the child, leaving it unable to touch the food or forcing it to spill it. The child can't move then and has nearly no active part in the feeding process. The only option it has is to turn its head away and, if that is made impossible, not to swallow and will spit or vomit. Spitting may cause parents to push further; they may start to hold their child's head and try to induce swallowing by stimulating its cheeks or even more intrusive measures. Eva Kerschischnik, physiotherapist in our team, may advise parents to put their child in a high chair opposite themselves and make eye contact. Sometimes eye contact may become too much of a stimulation for the child; in such cases, it must be changed again. The somewhat modern concept of a child taking part in its own nutrition could be compared to the movement toward women overseeing their body and their needs. This may be partly true for infants as well who should take part in their own decisions regarding whether and what to eat. A speech and language therapist (SLT) traditionally induces eating by stimulation around and in the oral cavity. This concept may be applicable to some disorders, and it may even work in some cases. In our concept the assessment of a baby's abilities is our goal. For instance, the baby might be able to swallow its own saliva. If that can be observed, then stimulating swallowing is unnecessary. If a baby can close its lips to make access to its mouth impossible, then opening its mouth by force shouldn't happen; it's intrusive. These are examples of why it is necessary to have a trained SLT on board.

After parents and children became tube dependent, a lot of psychological concerns arose. In the past, parents showing concern over tube weaning and even small changes in nutrition were transferred to a psychologist, child psychiatrist, or psychotherapist. Transfers tend to offend parents in need; they don't feel that they have a psychological disorder. Therefore, a member of the team should be responsible for anxiety and for overcoming traumas stemming from pregnancy or the after-birth period. Parents may be troubled by recollections from the intensive care or the feeling of guilt for a child needing oxygen support or being already endangered by everyday virus infections. Knowing this, we strongly recommend that every team member feels able and responsible for the needs of the parents and should be empathic. We met many doctors who turned away when a mother started to cry. They would clap on her shoulder and say unhelpful things like, "everything will turn out okay!" or "don't take it so serious. Other children we treat are far worse." Then they would whisper to the nurse, "arrange an appointment at our psychological department." We detest this kind of interaction. Sure, you don't have to be a psychotherapist on top of a pediatrician, but empathy doesn't require psychotherapeutic training only a humanitarian attitude. The instinct to get rid of parents showing signs of emotion is wrong. Having a psychologist and/or psychotherapist present shouldn't influence one's empathy. To have a psychologist in the team makes referrals unnecessary because problems are solved on the spot. Ultimately, it's necessary to combine different observations, speculations, and approaches in a well-functioning team.

Such a team follows the one rule that every team member deserves respect. Ancient hierarchies like in a monarchy or a cloister aren't helpful. Every approach, every piece of knowledge is as good as any other. The MD has no more to say than any other team member. This can be proven by watching some of the younger team members like interns. If they have input, they are not only listening to what the so-called experts have to say; then the team is most likely respectful. The team's functionality reflects the position of the families and especially the infants undergoing therapy. At the very least, it must be respected and take an active part in the process. That's the same situation as the infant who might have been an object and not the subject in therapy. In the end, every team member should try to have a holistic approach. For most questions everybody is competent. There are few questions, which can be answered only by a MD or a psychologist or a physiotherapist. Mostly, as in our ES, a question from parents or children can be answered by every team member. "Should my child eat?"—"Yes". "Is there anything it can't eat?" "Yes, very small children shouldn't start with an apple because they might choke" (all team members should know this from the interactive learning they have undergone or from the regularly held team meetings during the treatment). Multidisciplinary cooperation doesn't happen without commitment to one main idea: Nobody is worth more than any other person. It's not the MD who is most important due to international contacts or publications, nor is it the psychologist because he/she might feel competent for handling grief and sorrow; it's not the SLP who primarily knows how to change a child's attitude toward food; it's not the physiotherapist who mostly knows how to sit a handicapped child. All respect each other, their fields of knowledge, and learn from each other. If this moral cornerstone is the basis of working together, then respect toward the baby will be sincere and present.

4.3   Assessment of Oral Skills and Plans for Stimulating Them During Tube Weaning

The assessment and stimulation of oral skills may be seen as being easy, but we think that it requires a long time to master them in depth. We strongly advise to start with exclusive observation. There are a lot of recommendations and skills described in literature regarding when the assessment should be done.[1] Outstanding and wonderful work is done with babies during their stay in the NICU, mostly after they could be weaned from continuous oxygen support [4]. These studies show that early oral stimulation helps children to learn to eat when offered. Sadly, not enough of this is not done in hospitals, and we even saw sometimes the use of a lemon swab stemming from adult intensive care used with babies in order to stimulate them. It's highly aversive for them. The evaluation of oral stimulation may be done by measuring the amount eaten. Videofluoroscopy could also be a tool to assess babies swallowing competence but could only be used scientifically when performed for clinical reasons [5] due to ethical considerations. We are not sure whether videofluoroscopy is a good tool because it produces false results (saying that babies are unable to swallow or even aspirate liquid or food) if they cry. Even when a baby is not hungry, the test may show an inability to swallow. For the sake of the test, the velum palatinum is submitted to anesthesia using a spray, changing the function of the velum, and thus influencing the swallowing function. Relying only on this test for assessing the ability to drink would be wrong. Other tests measure intraoral pressure, ability of closing lips, the way the tongue moves (as seen using ultrasound), function of the muscles (like M. masseter) and/or the jaw joint, and even later the influence of the development of teeth and so forth. We strongly advise colleagues starting to learn more about the oral competence in children to observe! While watching, no intervention should be made. Later, an observer might want to reduce interferences of a tablet or a mobile phone used in order to distract the child while being fed. This shouldn't be done in children where parents claim that it can eat only when distracted.

A 4-year-old girl from Amsterdam would take long walks with her mother. She ate only when on the move or in a playground. The mother carried an open yoghurt in her hand easily accessible for little Ann. Ann would sometimes approach the little plastic tin and take a spoon full. They visited playgrounds and gardens, became an attraction for other visitors who talked with and about them, gave unrequested advice, and compared this feeding method to their own childhood or their parenting style. Ann would not eat a lot during these strolls. But it was still more than she ate at home. When observing Ann, one could see that she knew how to eat, to swallow,

---

[1] Lau C, Smith EO. A novel approach to assess oral feeding skills of preterm infants. *Neonatology*. 2011;100(1):64-70. doi:10.1159/000321987. Lau proposes a number of variables in order to perform an objective test to know what and how the preterm infant can and will eat. None of these variables respect the child as an active person, neither parents as supporters of the preterm child.

In another article (Lau C, Smith EO. Interventions to improve the oral feeding performance of preterm infants. Acta Paediatr. 2012 Jul;101(7):e269-74. doi: 10.1111/j.1651-2227.2012.02662.x. Epub 2012 Apr 5. PMID: 22404221.)

Lau et al. assess the sucking and swallowing abilities of the preterms. As the group of children is in the NICU while assessed their part in these experiments and observations is not reported. They are research-objects, which is good for research but quite opposite to our approach. On the other hand, we see these children when they have survived their impairments and outgrown the NICU. This leads to another understanding of the child's own role.

but she showed a lack of interest in food. In getting acquainted with parents, we learned that both parents had very little interest in food. None could cook, and the kitchen was used for coffee only. The story was even more interesting as Ann's grandparents had a restaurant when Ann's mother was a child. She was never allowed to be in the kitchen. Parents thought she could hurt herself and wanted her to advance in society becoming an academic. The reason for referring to this story is that it has been completely unnecessary to submit Ann to various tests like video-fluoroscopy and a swallow study. Observing and listening would have been sufficient.

A 5-year-old girl from Great Britain developed a rare mechanism when food was offered to her. Anisha produced enormous amounts of snot, which she processed like a bubble with her hands in a self-centered game. She could go on for hours. When mommy approached her with a spoon, she would produce snot and retreat to her own world. She suffered from a genetic disorder, her development was delayed, and she didn't speak and showed signs of autism spectrum disorder. But her orality was okay. She could swallow her saliva and her snot with ease. Behavioral therapy even included introduction of atypical neuroleptics had a tremendous effect, snot production was reduced, and Anisha could concentrate on food and start interacting with her mother and sister. Sadly enough, the recommended medication was not approved by MDs in Great Britain. Again, ENT assessment to find the reason for the enormous snot production was unnecessary. It was a bad habit more than a disease. Other tests turned out to be inconclusive as Anisha couldn't appropriately take part. Watching her somehow disgusting "game" allowed a diagnostic assumption and made a therapeutic attempt possible.

Barbora, a 5-month-old child from Czech Republic, was held on her mother's lap when being fed. It was Franziska's fourth child, and she was used to it. She did that with all her children. But Barbora was different. She choked a lot and stopped eating afterward. Putting B. on an upright pillow opposite her mother induced mutual interaction. The mother could see whether B would open her mouth and want more food for the first time. We could observe that B. was able to swallow. Our colleague being a SLP suspected recurrent aspirations happening, as had the team in Praha. But when B was on her reclining pillow during feeding, no aspiration could be seen and choking was rare. Therapeutic counseling was necessary as was intensive contacts to the other members of the team in Czech Republic.

The question of stimulating orality pre-eating when children are still on gavage is important [6]. It could be shown that it reduces the number of days in the NICU and helps the baby learn to eat. When a child doesn't want to eat or is seemingly unable, SLTs tend to stimulate in or around the mouth, the cheeks, and sometimes the collar. This may be helpful when a child is still on ventilation in a sedated mode. Afterward, it may be aversive or awkward. Our approach is different; we stimulate the child, its parents, and its environment. We create a food world, be it in our center in Graz, Austria, or via our telemedical online coaching (Netcoaching), where the child can stay at the family's home.

4.4   Encourage Self-Regulation and Stop External Control

In many cases when a child is on ENT, standardized tube formulas will be in the format of a pharmaceutical compound. It smells like a liquid drug. Parents keep all the tools necessary for gavage clean and in a special cupboard together with other medications. Thus, ENT is not only artificial but also smells and looks like it. This for the child its "food" is artificial. One could compare that to the evolution of money, what was once coins from copper, silver, and gold is now printed paper. Nowadays it has become virtual on smartphones and plastic cards. For children on ENS, their food doesn't induce appetite by its smell, its appearance, or the way it's presented. It doesn't smell as when onion is fried or the strong smell of cabbage fills the kitchen. Mother's hands are not sticky when she touches her baby, and the atmosphere a cake in the oven can induce cannot arise. Sometimes families prepare no meals on weekdays, or the family rarely eats cooked meals or uses pre-cooked meals from the supermarket. As everybody knows that the baby doesn't eat, nobody offers it food. Sometimes food is prepared for the baby but as the infant isn't hungry because the gavage filled it up, it doesn't eat.

Additionally, parents don't like their infant to play with food as they understandably don't want food to mess up the play corner of the child. A child on ENS has sometimes endured a long duration in an aseptic environment, and it and its parents are used to absolute hygiene and cleanliness. The smell of antiseptic solutions on the hands, which touched it, the odor of the whole ward, and the always clean industrially washed cloths, which were used of the baby—it made a hospital world without stinky smells from undisposed trash-bins and smelly armpits and of food which had been forgotten. Parents adjust to that and prefer their child to be neat and its clothing stain-free. We intervene by asking parents to create a "food world [7, 8]." Food should be available for a child which is mobile, all the time. It needn't be clean. A bar of chocolate is as good as sticky sweets or crunchy chips. Children should be allowed to carry food with them, keep it, and hold on to it. Use them as toys, crush it, and have it on the floor and on their bed covers, pillows, and chairs. As simple as our advice is, it can be incredibly hard to follow. Parents are mostly in despair because their child got stuck on a tube, but they still want to have cleanliness and order in their home.

I remember one exception from this rule from when Notube was still a travelling team, like a circus, we were offering an Eating-School in a youth hotel in Gnas, Styria. A Slovenian child, his mother, and its aunt also took part. The 3-year-old child took at breakfast 2–3 round Austrian rolls and kept them in her hands like dolls all day long. She never ate from them, but she didn't let them go. I observed that for 2 days. No change. The rolls became distorted throughout the day, and we tossed them in the garbage bin after dinner. They were the transition objects[2] of Svenia and protected her from taking part in meals or being molested with food by her family

---

[2] Like D. W. Winicott: The Child, the Family and the Outside World. London, 1964 described an object, which is in phantasy empowered by mother's emotions and can be used therefore by the child to cuddle and calm itself down before and during sleepiness.

and therapists. On the second day, I asked her mother Zonia to eat the rolls Svenia was holding in her hands. Svenia was upset, cried, slapped her mother, and ran away from her. Eventually when she approached her mother again, I asked Zonia to take a bite again. The rolls diminished, and the "food-resistant" Svenia recognized that the rolls were food and that food was for eating. She must have known before because she used it as a protection shield against intrusion and the pressure to eat while other food was on display. Svenia was a bright little girl: her next interaction was to offer parts of the rolls to her family, later to everybody. When therapists turned their heads away when Svenia offered, her mother imitated our behavior and Svenia tried to overcome our food resistance.

This kind of intervention is called a "paradox" intervention. For now, it's necessary to understand that a child transitioning needs confrontation with food as much as possible.

Transition from tube feeding to oral eating happens in these children at another age than it would in normally developing children. This is why adults don't see it as charming anymore. When a 6-month-old baby, transitions from breast milk to supplements one follows the steps of the learning process with empathy and joy. Even if it spills all content of its little dish on its high chair or on the floor, adults tend to find that cute. When a 5-year-old child achieves this, it looks abominable. When a child suffers from handicaps, it might even be disgusting. Spilling, drooling, munching, and spitting out pieces of food happen frequently. A lot of food is wasted and must be thrown away. Our food world may seem disgusting to adults; in kindergarten children are educated not to spill, not to waste, and to learn polite table manners. Conversely, for children learning to eat in and after an ENS at any age, the learning shouldn't include table manners or to learn to like "healthy food." It's the learning child's decision what and how it starts to eat.

We observed an enormous variation in what children like and want. Some would start eating ice cream, some sausage, and some popsicles; others munched marshmallows, usually spitting out most of it. Parents should also eat while the child does so. It's a challenge. Often the floor or the table is covered with food and its remnants covered with saliva. Sweet and savory food may be mixed, emitting a strange odor. The child may be covered with chocolate, and it may be smeared around its mouth. Stains of all different kinds of food may be on the child's clothes. We ask parents not to use bibs because they tend to arouse bad memories and are uncomfortable. This leads to garments full of stains, urging mothers to change them after every meal. Mealtimes can't be kept clean with children while transitioning. The child may grab a bite while on the run or doesn't want to sit or behave. Essentially, a child and its family taking our advice seriously may never be clean during the process of learning to eat.

Self-regulation requires the empowerment of the child and a reduction of the parental influence over food and its intake. We support this process by asking parents to use an online intake protocol: all intakes, be it by gavage or orally, are listed and documented by them and recognized by us. Thus, we take over the control of some of the parent's daily burden, being available twice daily all year. In a psychoanalytical model, one could say we take the role of the superego, thus liberating parents from their responsibility a bit. The child may use its own path and speed. If food stops being offered or a parent is too invasive with a spoon or any other device, the child may start to open its mouth or leave it closed.

We as counselors look for specific problems like dehydration and/or obstipation, which both may be caused by a lack of fluid. The child, who is left with reduced gavage, may start looking for liquid or food itself. It may take a few days (this period may be shortened if nearly no intervention be it physical or verbal happens). The transition needs patience, although parents will be concerned that their child may starve or be subjected to dehydration; MDs may have the same apprehensions. It's notable that oral intake doesn't start right away. Weaning protocols, which request that oral intake compensates for gavage completely from the first day on, tend to use very little steps in reducing the amount of gavage (and maybe the transition attempt fails because the child adapts to the new "diet"). They may reintroduce more tube feeds when nutritional goals are not met, or weight loss starts, when a child caught a cold, or anesthesia requirements, etc. If an intravenous drip is given, we prefer a nutritious fluid instead of reintroducing a temporary tube. The child leads the way into oral eating; we are merely the bystanders. We try to put parents (and our colleagues) in the same position. As little intervention as possible, distant admirers of the child's path—that's the right way to allow a child to learn to eat.

4.5   Step Back and Just Observe What Happens

This applies to all adults concerned. We merely look at, even admire, a child learning to eat, how it approaches scary substances, which may smell or be sticky or dissolve in one's hand. It can be very exciting. Even the behavior of the parents changes in these moments. The child cannot know why. Perhaps the other adults induced that change or the people from the computer to whom the parents speak frequently. Be it how it may—parents are different. Eating on the floor is permissible, not forbidding spilling or taking food to the sofa, which used to be out of the question. Interventions around food and eating nearly stopped. The child may behave the way it wants. It may lick, munch, spit, or throw food with an expression of joy into the garbage bin. On the other hand, parents are not allowed to do that. Perhaps they want to play the same game and throw "good" food in the bin as well. We don't ask parents to do so, for it works only when it is authentic. Parents needn't be actors. If they hate throwing food in the bin, they shouldn't pretend to. It's challenging enough to stay encouraging, serene, confident, calm, and agreeable. We treated Ossip, a 3-year-old, who wouldn't eat at all. His mother lived a vegan life; his father ate non-vegan food, but only outside the house. Maria, his mother, was very strict with food. It had to be the best of the best, organically grown and harvested in a nearby farm, which she visited weekly. Ossip didn't take part in the whole buying, cooking, and eating process nor did his father. They behaved like carnivores in a world of plant-eaters. They refrained as would lions or cheetahs do when offered vegetables. When the family took part in our Eating-School, Oskar started drinking high-calorie drinks and eating sausages when peeled. At home, he stopped eating and stayed with his drinks.

One could call that being on ENS as he didn't eat solid foods. Parents felt that this way of sustaining himself had no future. We met them in a café, where we all had cappuccinos, Maria's with rice milk. Ossip longed for a drink. Marguerite offered hers to him. He licked the milk foam from the top of the cup. He did so with all four coffees. From that moment on, Ossip had 8–10 coffee foam cups/day. He switched from Nutricia's Nutrini drink, a highly balanced drink, to milk foam. At that point one may think that Ossip could be suffering from an autism spectrum disorder (ASD) as he could barely adapt to changes, but diagnosis of ASD can only be made after entering school. He could detect facial expressions, spoke German very well, and related to his parents as well as to other people. Only regarding food, he was quite strict. We assumed that his mother was as strict as he was; he was projecting her. We could have asked mother to have meat or sausage at home. It would be nearly as impossible for her as it would be for a Hindi family. We approached the situation with more care; we asked his father to take his son out sometimes for a bite of fast food, which is offered in a town like Vienna at every corner: sausage, kebab, meat, rolls, cakes, and sweets. Gradually Ossip shifted his food intake to moments away from home. It was only then that his mother told us that she never liked food. When it became necessary to feed her own child, she tried her best but felt like a failure. This is a point where we needed to step back. The mother's story should be addressed in psychotherapy. Unfortunately, she had undergone psychotherapy before and didn't like it. She felt that she was blamed for all Ossip endured. She felt guilty, but psychotherapy didn't help to improve the situation, and she felt even worse.

Being a food therapist, one must understand that every remark which indicates that parents are responsible for the trouble should be taken seriously. Be cautious, observe, and don't make any quick assumptions. Be aware that nearly all parents wish the best for their children; criminals and abusers rarely appear in our clinics. One may share one's observations, but they shouldn't contain any judgment. Parents feel judgment even if their therapist doesn't intend it. Parents quickly think that one is going to propose to them a new way of interaction when reflecting one's observations. They want to obey but are anxious and resistant against change. One's approach must be as tentative as possible. The therapist should hold back and speak rarely. How can one be recognized as a "friendly observer"? By not smiling all the time, nor nodding one's head all the time, but by joining the child and its family, being calm and interested.

One shouldn't approve or deny what one sees, it's not required to judge children or their parents' performances. My (PS) psychoanalytic teacher Ekstein [9] used to say: "We have to change from urgency to time." As much urgency parents feel ("The Eating-School lasts only a fortnight!" or "If it doesn't cooperate—what shall we do?" "Can't you push him/her?"), as much stress they have, instinctively they want to hand over some of their stress to the therapist; the therapist should never be stressed. Changing the way a child eats is in itself not a stressful task. One has a lot of time. Parents tend to impose stress, pointing to the side effects of gavage or malnutrition. Other circumstances, such as upcoming changes in parent's jobs or holidays, may lead to stress on their side. A therapist should never be a part of that. A friendly observer should be interested, laughing, and watching and show emotions if truly felt but shouldn't get stressed as much as possible.

4.6   Refrain from Pessimistic Judgments If a Child Drinks Water Without Difficulties

In our experience, very good and highly respected institutions may sometimes decide that a child is not able or allowed to eat or to drink at all. "Nil by mouth!" is the verdict, which leads to ENS. The diagnosis, which is the reason for that judgment is called "silent aspiration," mostly without clinical signs of aspiration, like coughing or recurrent pneumonia. In children with inborn or postpartum problems, like pulmonary diseases such as a bronchopulmonary dysplasia due to an underdeveloped lung, which made long-lasting auxiliary ventilation necessary, or a child born with a diaphragmatic hernia, which inhibited the development of one lung, medical teams tend to be even more cautious. This is understandable and we respect that. At Notube we try to get in touch with the teams to discuss their insights when parents apply, in order to wean their child, and we don't pay too much attention to the anxiety of doctors and SLPs. As mentioned already, the results of a videofluoroscopy and a swallow test using X-ray can often be inconclusive when the baby cried. If so, it may aspirate when fed while crying. Nobody can eat and swallow safely when too excited or even crying. I (PS) remember a 11.2 km run I made back in 2012 through the Plabutsch Tunnel in Graz, Austria. The refurbished tunnel was offered to lunatics for a once in a lifetime run. Before finishing, a nice young lady offered me a dry cookie made from sugar, egg yolk, and almonds—very dry. I took it into my mouth, choked while jogging the remaining path, and felt like I would suffocate. Compare a baby resisting a meal being constrained in a machine. Intra-abdominal pressure will change tremendously while circled around due to crying, holding air back, and exhaling fast. The same is true for the videofluoroscopy. A child is kept on the mother's lap, and the device is put through the child's nose. Then the reflecting agent is installed. Children who didn't learn to eat may not open their mouth, keeping their lips shut with force. Already inserting the liquid might induce furious crying.

When children taste the substance almost none like it. The ENT doctor may try to calm the baby and its mother while being themself stressed. This attempt rarely succeeds. In the end a lot of these tests are performed while patients are bothered so they don't swallow. The substance runs down the pharynx without swallowing. As the epiglottis doesn't close clearly, aspiration can't be excluded. The result reads as follows: "A tendency to aspirate can't be excluded. Further tests may be necessary in 3-month time." One could call these results inconclusive. It doesn't help the decision of the feeding team whether a given child is allowed to eat orally or not. To stay on the safe side, doctors often recommend not to start offering food orally. Sometimes the child doesn't want to eat; sometimes it starts eating by itself.

Sometimes, when no clinical aftereffects happen, doctors give in. We strongly advise colleagues not to express and permit any negative judgments concerning shortcomings or inabilities of any sort when the child is in the room. We seemingly react neutrally when parents tell us the medical problems of the child. We overdo this sometimes and tend to overlook "real" diseases. But how would you start treating a child suffering from leukemia or after a kidney transplant receiving immunosuppressive medication? How would you start with children where scientific literature shows "evidence" that they will never learn to eat, like Pierre-Robin and CHARGE syndrome? Would you be strong enough to risk the transition in a 3-year-old infant who is scheduled for his/her next heart operation already in a year? Would you risk weight loss? What's about all those children we treated suffering from kidney insufficiency receiving medication, which is known to taste bitter (like spironolactone)? These obstacles were enormous for us and still are. Seeing children learning to eat even when their lifespan is very short due to genetic disorders like trisomy 18, some months was more than rewarding. The child had another year to live and enjoyed food and eating very much. Parents felt that they had a nearly normal child and had fun with each other. Feeding was adding interaction and family functioning. For sure one could have concentrated on the missing abilities of the child instead.

4.7   Follow the Child But Respect the Opinions of the Mother, Father, Family, and Team

For us, the child is our partner in the weaning process. We know that the parents are very important too. In our Netcoaching program, the first and only partners are parents who pay for the service and interact with us. We can observe the child in the videos the parents tape, choose, and upload on our platform. Nevertheless, it's a video curated by parents in a situation they created and controlled. We don't advise our readers to watch the baby continuously and ask it what it wants and how it is going to perform. Our focus on the child is more like an opposition to common pediatrics where doctors and therapists concentrate on the parents while dealing with their infant. An everyday scene in the emergency room of the university hospital we used to witness for nearly 30 years was as follows: Child and mother would enter the room and sit opposite the doctor. The mother answers questions like "Since when is your child ill?" or "Are there any chronic diseases?" or "have they had fever?". Meanwhile a nurse is putting the infrared thermometer into the child's ear—it may start to cry already. The child didn't speak until this moment and may not speak at all subsequently. It recognized the situation as frightening where his/her mother speaks with the doctor and eventually with the nurses. The child doesn't feel like the subject of the assessment or the therapeutic measures taken but rather as an object subject to the will of others. When later asked to swallow a pill, it may not only reject it due to anxiety or inability to swallow but because it wasn't addressed as a subject before. It may happen that a schoolchild may be overlooked although everybody knows that this child is able to speak about its symptoms. We were never able to change this attitude. When in charge we could behave differently, but the price was high. We were seen as the "psychos" doing things differently, extending the timespan in the emergency room putting its main functionality at stake.

When assessing a child who comes to us online or in real life, we address the child first. We offer some food on a little table or tablet which can be reached by the child in most cases. We don't offer food, which might be harmful like apple pieces or carrots. When parents start to interject (mostly because they are stressed or assume the doctor's time is limited), we try to keep them back. We try to get in touch with the child even when it sits on their mother's or any caregiver's lap. We don't approach the child in a childish manner but in a respectful way as we do with parents. When caretakers try to get rid of the child by asking, for example, the partner to hold the child so that the mother can speak more frankly, we withdrew. We listen, and we comment seldomly. Be respectful. Marguerite tends to interfere by asking clarifying questions and tries to orientate herself in the logic of the parents. Ronny prefers to "go with the flow." For him it's not necessary to understand everything. As the child doesn't come into the day clinic for an operation it's not necessary to know everything on the first day. Symptoms may evolve; disease-related questions shall be addressed; for the first encounter the appearance of the child may be sufficient.

Both ways have as much merit as each other. There may be more interactional models used. All are as good as any other. We think that only two main points should be remembered: (1) don't forget to address the child; and (2) be vigilant; make it possible that you see, observe, and feel, i.e., tune in. The first contact needs a feeding team, which is aware of the special situation the patient and the family are in. It's like a wedding or a funeral: for the priest it's their normal everyday job. For the couple, it should be a very special day in their life. The same is true for funerals: for the family of the person, which passed away, it's a special day, which will be remembered. The role of the priest (or whomever) is to make it special. This needs a lot of attention and awareness. It needs some knowledge of the specific case, but more than that it needs attention to detail, interest, and a gentle emotional tact. It's not only about the facts, but rather it's about creating mutual trust and understanding. Assumptions are made unwillingly on both sides. Be cautious to present yourself in a way eliciting assumptions like "this a classical MD," or "this doctor has no clue, they didn't prepare for our meeting," or "they are only interested in our child and not what we have endured."

The same is true for the doctor him-/herself. Assumptions made because specific clothing can't be omitted but try to control them. Not every mother clothed in a homely soft style is poor or uneducated. Not every father using his mobile phone frequently is uninterested. We remember a grandfather from Netherlands joining his daughter in an Eating-School who traded interests on his IWatch. When we knew him better, he exclaimed sometimes what he had earned, or lost. In the beginning respect was not so easily obtained as we felt disturbed and would have liked to ask him to refrain from "playing" with his watch. As trust kicked in, we learned that he can listen while trading. The rest of the family, namely, his wife, his daughter, and his son-in-law, were accustomed to that style. He is a loving and supportive grand-father knowing that his grandsons suffer from a genetically transferred kidney disease which their mother, his daughter, passed on to them on. To know that isn't easy at all. Perhaps trading helps to cope.

4.8   If the Process Is Stuck, Analyze Possible Aversive Variables

This subchapter is tricky because it asks for self-reflection. For example, a 3-year-old child comes to your clinic on total ENS using a PEG. According to a protocol, one reduces the amount of gavage swiftly approx. by 30% in 2 days. Nothing happens. All attempts to offer food are futile. The consequences on doctors and even parent's side are clear, reducing the gavage further. Nothing changes, the child starts to lose weight, and parents get stressed. Sometimes the child may get a little disturbed and cry more often. More talks between the therapeutic team and parents take place. Unintentionally, on a subconscious level, every party blames the other. When in that situation, one must take a step back. Never blame the parents even when they start offering food all the time. They learn it in a hard way from their child when it shows signs of resistance they try to ignore. It turns its head away when offered food, cries when parents start to force food into its mouth, and perhaps vomits after being fed. The choices available are at least (a) indulge in an attempt of force feeding; (b) enhance the amount of gavage again, wait if possible in 1–2 days, and start reducing again; (c) submit parents to further "learning" by adding appointments with the SLP and/or psychotherapist; or wait and see. A lot of other "interventions"'could be made. In all cases nobody should be held accountable for the problem. Perhaps the team hasn't understood the infant well enough, or perhaps something in the room disturbed the child, which hindered it from learning to eat. I remember an acoustically oversensitive child. The noises, the chatter, the clinging of dishes, and the sound from the kitchen was simply too much. And MD who was herself sound-sensitive recognized that Jonah started to eat only at the end of the play picnic, which he tried to leave till the last 45 min. Only after most people left, and the kitchen was closed and members of the team started to clean up, then Jonah ate. It helped him when his parents were available but concentrated on other things like preparing to leave. They had lost interest and gave up. This helps in numerous situations because the focus isn't any more on the child and it becomes free to explore. Be cautious here; don't intervene. When intervening right away, one could disturb Jonah's solution. Don't tell parents that they should feed Jonah while at home. This won't work. Parents will again concentrate on Jonah's eating; maybe they will even start to offer food again. The food will be spiced with stress, expectations, and hope. Instead, one should wait for the next rounds or any other interaction between parents and team to point out that Jonah found a solution. He learnt to cope with his appetite or even huger sensations within the given system. After having observed Jonah's solution, we tried noise-reducing earphones on him, which he tossed away. We allocated him one parent at a time in a room where they were alone, but it didn't work, because the caregiver concentrated on Jonah and his eating again. In the end we found a solution for Jonah and the rest of the attending clients. Whenever Jonah showed signs of distress, he could leave the play picnic room, take a little stroll within the Eating-School, and come back afterward mostly by himself. This happened in the beginning 3–5 times per hour. Nobody cared; nobody was stressed anymore. Jonah travelled in and out perhaps waiting for the situation in which he could eat. Sometimes he went (before COVID-19 regulations) to the cook's kitchen to which only certain personnel are allowed. But as food was already delivered and the kitchen would be cleaned after lunch, our cook always had time for Jonah. Once Jonah asked for a bite of something, he got it. Without parents or therapists, he munched on it. Mr. Kruger, the chef, felt tickled pink that he was Jonah's successful therapist.

4.9   Giving Up on a Child with a Potential to Transit to Oral Feeding Is a Failure

A lot of parents visit us, or come to our clinic, or use our service electronically, after already having made some attempts at tube weaning. They may have been in a reha-bilitation center for weeks or even months without success. Sometimes parents point out that it was defined as success that their child doesn't vomit any more when being confronted with food. Sometimes the child learnt to attend a family meal without crying. In other cases, the attempt of tube weaning was made at home under the guidance of a SLT or a psychologist. Maybe the child started to open its mouth when asked to do so. Be aware at first: never ever make any negative or critical remarks about attempts done elsewhere, concerning ideas and therapeutic measure-ments. Even if one detests these measures, like we do concerning force feeding and/ or restraining a child in its high chair for the sake of eating, one must be cautious. First it may have been necessary at the time, when we still didn't know the child; second, it's like spilled milk, declaring what we would have done otherwise is infan-tile. We would enjoy the bliss of the moment when we feel superior but pay the price of acquiring an enemy or turning a whole institution into a hostile land for us. I remember us doing so when we were younger and travelling through the world to make tube weaning a method used by pediatricians as well as child psychiatrists. We felt great; we were young after all. But we lost New Zealand as well as Australia as possible customers because we showed them our "superiority." Having said that, the next step must be done. When we get stuck trying to wean a child from its tube, we must start from scratch. We must rethink our diagnostic working model; we have to discuss the therapeutic interventions made and to reflect our interactions with the whole family. A mother came from Frankfurt, Germany, where she lived with her twins and her husband. Both parents were bankers. The mother moved out of daily trading and became a convenience manager, while the father was online trading 8–10 h/day. He came home to sleep, while Mother was with her genetically identical twins attending the Eating-School. One girl was weaker, both being born in the 26th week of gestational age. This girl had some developmental delays and was on fully ENS, while her sibling could move perfectly and eat. Mother came originally from a farm in Styria, Austria, maybe that was one reason why she chose our clinic. She was brought up a farm girl; she was prepared to do everything which her children needed. After 1 week when our client, the weaker twin, hadn't learned anything, we asked the father to come from Frankfurt to attend our school as well. I add sometimes to my request a small sentence that if one can't leave the office on behalf of a child in need for a certain time, then it doesn't matter in the end whether the person is in their job or not. No hope exists for advancement if an intermission of work is nearly impossible.

Father came on a Friday and stayed until Tuesday. He didn't know why we asked him in and what we wanted him to do. We explained that his wife and his child needed his attention. He started to explain how stressful his job was, how much he invests and gains only for the sake of his family and so forth. Some people think that they are irreplaceable and suppose that they work not for their own ego but for their family. We listened carefully and answered that his family and our team needed his help. "What and how?" was the reply. We answered by dealing with the "healthy" brother, with the same attention and emotion of his wife and by visiting his wife's family on Sunday. He obliged. To his surprise he was a big help. It was even surprising for him that his absence was a source of constant drain for his wife; that she was missing him not only as a father but as a husband; that his attempt to make a career was his wish, nobody else needed that; and so forth. Thus couple functions were strengthened as was rearing. Before both parents had told us that he wouldn't be able to come to Graz. If it would have been for money, for an inheritance, or a funeral, it would have been made possible. So why not for the sake of supporting the therapy? Why not help one's child when it needs it most? Why wait until mother and children come home having endured a failure? Never take circumstances or impossibilities for granted. Think of the impossible as an obstacle and no more. Eventually think of movies where aliens try to invade the earth trying to erase mankind. Suddenly all wars cease, and humanity responds as one group wanting to survive. The same is true for our fairy tale of tube weaning. When we feel that we can't win, we have to rethink everything, which might hinder the child. If allocated, one should try to change it.

4.10 Trying New Approaches Again and Again Is Not a Failure

When one thinks they have done everything and nothing worked, one should try a new approach. When we were trained as psychotherapists, new ideas were born in the late 1960s and 1970s of the last century. "Paradox intervention" was one of them. We had frequent contact, about twice daily, with a mother online. Her 4-year-old boy was a picky eater.[3] He ate a very small variety of nutrients: a specific yoghurt, rolls without butter or anything else, he drank one brand of cacao, and sometimes he would eat French fries from McDonalds. The mother tried everything. Given that such an eating disorder can only emerge when a codependent person is available who is frightened that the child may starve and supports its pickiness, we tried as much as possible to change the mother's habits. None of us changed, nobody moved, neither child, nor mother, nor us. We gave advice like "don't buy that specific yoghurt," and Clark's mother did what she was told. Clark had no yoghurt for a while. He ate more rolls and less protein. We all were completely stuck. One day his mother wrote in her ticket, which is the online message area during the Netcoaching process: "Clark eats only rolls now, he lacks supplements, essential fatty- and amino acids. What now?" It was not a good day for our team. Most of us allocated to that client (a psychologist, an eat therapist, and a MD) were emotionally done with Clark. So, the simple answer was: "If he decides to do so, let him." Normally we would have tried new ways, creating new environments for Clark and his mother or we would take a step back and offer him "his yoghurt" again. Clark's mother was not at all happy with our answer. She was offended and didn't answer at all. We feared that we lost her but felt subconsciously a sense of relief. We had done what we had asked his mother to do for a long time: we didn't support her overanxious and overinvolved motherhood anymore. After a few days, it might have been a week, a new message came in: "Clark stopped nearly completely on rolls and his daily cacao. He asked for a bite from the sandwich I ate!" This was a new start. Mother saw for the first time that Clark was not prepared to risk his life, to sacrifice it for his special preferences and to his anxiety, but to try something new instead.

There is always hope. Sometimes, especially children like those suffering from a Down syndrome and others suffering from similar diseases which lead to stubbornness of the child might be stronger than any therapist. Perhaps the child doesn't know what it wants but what it doesn't want seems clear. Heart failure and its operation, the big tongue, etc.—all that and a lot more is blamed to be the cause for the food resistance in these children. On the other hand, there are a lot of children with Down syndrome who eat and drink normally. We found that there is no point becoming as stubborn as the child to impose one's will over the handicapped child. We remember treating a child from Auckland, New Zealand, now 19 years old who came for treatment to Graz when he was 12. His mother had to leave her job when Jakob was born. He needed her full attention. Married to a filmmaker, and being herself a TV producer, the couple led a jet-set life. This changed dramatically as Jakob underwent two heart operations, stayed in intensive care the first year of his life, and needed his mother in the hospital and, from then on, all day long. Eventually they divorced, Jakob's father met another woman, and income dropped dramatically. Jakob developed very well receiving all possible support, but he didn't learn to eat and needed a JPEG (jejunal percutaneous gastrostomy) for nutrition. He was

---

[3] "Picky eating" is a disturbance, which is no diagnosis in the DSM in the year 2022. DSM is the US-American manual for psychiatric disorders—It describes an eating problem, formerly known in psychoanalysis as "Essideosynkrasie," in which the child eats only strictly defined products, mostly not more than 5–10 different items.

accustomed to it. When he became hungry, he pointed to the JPEG and mother complied. We reduced his feeds swiftly, which were at the age of 12 like 1400 mL/day. He knew that all the adults wanted him to start eating, but he didn't. The fortnight our Eating-School lasts passed by uneventfully. Mother and her parents, who came to help her, decided to stay for a holiday in Europe and booked the next term, which was scheduled after 21 days. Jakob had made in between no development in his eating skills. We decided to put him again on full ENS using his JPEG. He regained the intermediate weight loss and became friendly, even smiling at the next Eating-School. This time we decided to end all gavage. His JPEG received only 3 × 15 mL/day so that it wouldn't clog. Jakob was very thirsty and hungry. We explained to him why. He understood me, hugged me, and observed me while I was drinking and eating. He was very close and touchy with me. He nearly abandoned his mother during that period. She received daily psychological support. Jakob didn't eat or drink. It was a warm summer. Anxieties arose; dehydration became an issue especially because of his heart condition. We didn't change anything; nothing by ENS was the verdict. Jakob eventually became weak; he used to lie on the floor and look around but moved very little. His mother would bring him in with a pram to the Eating-School. We asked his mother to bring him in and leave for a walk nearby, just for an hour or so. She started crying uncontrollably. Jakob saw his mother's anguish, felt her pain. Perhaps to calm her down, to soothe her, he drank a glass of water. Starting with little sips, going on until he finished the plastic glass. Then his mother broke out in laughter, and Jakob did the same. Both couldn't stop laughing. They left for the lunch break and from then on Jakob decided to drink and eat. Perhaps he did so to make his mother happy; we will never know. Seven years later, we visited Jakob in Auckland. He hugged us; he stayed close to us. We went out for lunch. He ordered French fries for himself and some fish. He ate his whole plate. His grandmother invited us for that lovely dinner on a green hill in Auckland. This is to say never give up. Try again; do the most absurd things; behave unpredictably. Most important: stay tuned in and perform your work with vigor.

4.11   In Rare Cases the Transition to Oral Feeding Might Fail But May Work Out Later

To end this chapter, which might be seen as an introduction to a new way of perspective, bear in mind that all we have written so far may be wrong as well. Paradoxical thoughts as well as paradox interventions are a crucial phenomenon when dealing with children whose only ability is to refrain to say "No!" and to turn away when food is offered. In the assessment process, which is obligatory before any treatment may start, we see the most beautiful homes, the best equipped kitchens, and rooms which have been furnished to a child's needs and liking as much as possible. Amidst these wonderful homes, we would see a father or a mother offering a spoon full of baby food or soup or something else to their child who would turn its head away. Here the parent may become more intrusive for the sake of the recording, which in turn may induce crying in the child. The recording lasts 60–90 s because uploading is limited. At home this scene could last hours; parents may introduce a device on which the child may look at movies or anything that distracts and reduces resistance. Sometimes we are lucky. We observe the same child drinking its cup of water by itself without parents involved. Sometimes a film is sent to us where a child takes a bite of something. In all these cases, we are more or less sure that the child will be able to eat.

But sometimes we see a child unable to take a sip of clear water. Coughing after it drinks the water, retching, and clinging for air. As if it felt like being suffocated. Even then we ask for a swallow test and a consent from the local SLP. We treated an 8-month-old child from the Netherlands. Their father was a soldier, and mother an artist, and made for a very good-looking couple. Syrena was a very small child. When we first met her at the entrance of the Eating-School, she gasped, inhaled deeply, and had a hard time swallowing her saliva, eventually retching. The big soldier could nearly keep her in his hands; she was like a fish trying to break free. As if saying "Good Morning!" I asked the parents to take the NG tube out right away. Afterward Syrena could breathe more easily, and even more surprisingly Syrena liked food, drank even from a baby bottle and sustained herself by oral eating from this very moment on. Everybody was happy. In the second week she started to vomit. Between 10 min after eating up to an hour, she would vomit everything she had eaten. She would vomit like a spring. Without crying or showing signs of distress, she would get rid of her intake, being as friendly and happy as before. At first, we suspected gastroenteritis, but none of the other participants of the term had any symptoms. In a home visit at the flat her parents had rented for 14 days, we asked her parents if we could try to feed Syrena. She showed signs of hunger and we wanted to try. Syrena drank in one go her whole bottle. She looked satisfied afterward. We talked with her parents, and the situation was relaxed. Suddenly Syrena became a spring. The whole milk sprung out of her and covered the sofa she was laid on. We were desperate as were the parents. We thought of any pediatric diagnosis like pylorostenosis, any enteral obstruction, disorders of motility, and so forth. We transferred her to the children's surgical department in Graz, Austria. Telling them what we observed, asking them not to give us a simple answer, subsequently we failed. The doctor on duty decided that Syrena was suffering from an infectious dysentery and instructed parents to give her enough fluid. We were ashamed of the doctors in whom we gave our trust. We felt sorry for Syrena and her parents and were afraid that they would become angry with us, but nothing bad happened. Her father, accustomed to obeying, and her mother who was simply desperate complied. They gave Syrena as much fluid as she could take and drove home. In the online aftercare program, her vomiting, which had impressed us so much, ceased. We will never know whether there was a temporary obstruction or an enteral infection as the colleague suspected. Whatever it was, Syrena drank and ate but unfortunately didn't gain much weight. Later, she underwent surgery with the placement of a PEG. Sadly enough, it didn't help her as well. We also must be humble to accept such courses, where a lack of distinct communication on many levels most probably hid a specific detail which we were blind to see and react to.

References

1. Bos AF, van Loon AJ, Martijn A, van Asperen RM, Okken A, Prechtl HF. Spontaneous motility in preterm, small-for-gestational age infants. I. Quantitative aspects. Early Hum Dev. 1997;50(1):115–29. https://doi.org/10.1016/s0378-3782(97)00096-0. PMID: 9467697.
2. Puchalski M, Hummel P. The reality of neonatal pain. Adv Neonatal Care. 2002;2(5):233–44; quiz 245-7. PMID: 12881937.
3. Kamen RS. Impaired development of oral-motor functions required for normal oral feeding as a consequence of tube feeding during infancy. Adv Perit Dial. 1990;6:276–8. PMID: 1982825.
4. Rocha AD, Moreira ME, Pimenta HP, Ramos JR, Lucena SL. A randomized study of the efficacy of sensory-motor-oral stimulation and non-nutritive sucking in very low birthweight infant. Early Hum Dev. 2007;83(6):385–8. https://doi.org/10.1016/j.earlhumdev.2006.08.003. Epub 2006 Sep 18. PMID: 16979854.
5. Moon CW, Jung HG, Cheon HJ, Oh SM, Ki YO, Kwon JY. Verification of reliability and validity of the feeding and swallowing scale for premature infants (FSSPI). Ann Rehabil Med. 2017;41(4):631–7. https://doi.org/10.5535/arm.2017.41.4.631. Epub 2017 Aug 31. PMID: 28971048; PMCID: PMC5608671.
6. Lessen BS. Effect of the premature infant oral motor intervention on feeding progression and length of stay in preterm infants. Adv Neonatal Care. 2011;11(2):129–39. https://doi.org/10.1097/ANC.0b013e3182115a2a. PMID: 21730902.
7. Dunitz-Scheer M, Wilken M, Walch G, Schein A, Scheer P. Wie kommen wir von der Sonde los?! [How do we get rid of the tube?]. Kinderkrankenschwester. 2000;19(11):448–56. German. PMID: 11271003.
8. Dunitz-Scheer M, Levine A, Roth Y, et al. Prevention and treatment of tube dependency in infancy and early childhood. ICAN Infant Child Adolesc Nutr. 2009;1(2):73–82. https://doi.org/10.1177/1941406409333988.
9. Ekstein R. The language of psychotherapy. Benjamins, Amsterdam; 1989.

The Composition and Task of the Feeding Team

In the past two to three decades, some pediatric hospitals have made efforts to install interdisciplinary feeding teams to address tube maintenance and dependency. In some cases, this originates from a sense of institutional responsibility and is conducted by the specific health systems superior professionals. In other cases, such activities represent more of a compensatory task to service worried parents asking for more or better support. In any case, having a feeding team should address feeding issues in a systematic way. A feeding team needs more than the desire to help or mere minimal interest in the topics of food and irregular feeding. As eating and drinking are so basic, everyone feels that they are an expert, ready to give advice based on common sense, personal experience, intuition, and instinct. This can work and has been an effective transgenerational method of raising infants for thousands of years. But advice from relatives may also prove wrong as Justus Liebig [1] points out already in his eighteenth-century writings, "grandmothers and even midwives told young mothers to feed their baby using cow or even goat-milk. The cow milk led to severe malnutrition, whereas the goat-milk killed some babies due to anemia."

Today, there is extensive training for dieticians, dietician counselors, and the vast subspecialty of pediatric gastroenterology dealing mainly with a sufficient supply of minerals, trace elements, vitamins, and other food-related topics.

The primary team involved initially in the topics of tube indication and placement (nurse, surgeon, specialized pediatrician, ENT doctor and SLP, OT, nutritionist, psychologist) of any child would also be the best team to monitor and manage the child and its needs *after* tube placement and *through the phases* of tube maintenance and eventually tube weaning/aftercare. Unfortunately, this necessity is rarely understood from the perspective of the young patients and tends to be integrated into healthcare systems which doesn't put doctors into positions of being responsible of ENS aftercare. Even specialized rehabilitation centers offer medical advice mostly by external counselors only on request in order to cut costs. A specialist for tube placement will rarely see the child he operated on, apart from surgical aftercare. The doctor therefore might not even be aware and recognize troubles or side

© The Author(s), under exclusive license to Springer Nature Switzerland AG 2022
M. Dunitz-Scheer, P. J. Scheer, *Child-led Tube-management and Tube-weaning*, https://doi.org/10.1007/978-3-031-09090-5_5

effects besides leaking at the place of insertion or recurrent vomiting. We suggest that ENS must be recognized clearly as a distinct medical intervention (like any medication or any medical device necessary) and ongoing guidance should be obligatory.

Gastroenterologists tend to indulge in "talking" about feeding issues to families much more readily—and often don't have the same patience to listen to the mothers—than psychologists or psychotherapists would discuss their laymen insights on gut function. We were asked numerous times to offer advice to colleagues in different countries, who felt exhausted and began to hate non-compliant parents. When parents were curious or resistant toward the doctor's proposals, colleagues acted surprised, rather than asking parents to explain their own thoughts and beliefs. They tried to persuade parents to "do better" by increasing expectations about weight gain, sometimes using threats or even blackmailing them. Instead of leaning back and listening, they felt the need to make parents trust in their knowledge based primarily on the fact that the issue was "only feeding." When therapeutic methods were evaluated and found to be unhelpful or even harmful, doctors remained stubborn regarding their own practices. Science still has the authority like the church, and they were its priests. Disagreement was abolished and criticism not allowed. Doctors felt that their arguments had to win. It was no longer a question of supporting parents to help their child but became a question of victory or defeat.

Psychotherapists and gastroenterologists training in skills outside of their own is scarce; a "psychosomatic" thinking and specific education and training on feeding issues exist in very few countries. We recommend that in a feeding team, pediatric *and* psychodynamic knowledge should be present. A psychosomatically oriented doctor must have undergone a pediatric postdoc education as well as a psychotherapeutic training. Only then a MD can cover most of the presenting problems. Within the team additional psychological and dietician knowledge should be available as well as other a good portion of self-criticism and the willingness to try new ideas.

Meanwhile, food marketing uses highly suggestive and aggressive means of advertising. Food companies insinuate that only their product will make any baby thrive. This is of course not true, but modern standardized food is based on scientific research. If applied, it makes sure children's needs are met even when using ENS exclusively. Unfortunately, many centers offer guidance by dietitians or SLPs only, and their impact on decision-making is limited regarding the amount and/or content of ENS. The power and authority lie in the MD's hands, who may not be available when families come for feeding matters or even wanting to transition from ENS to orality. Without the position of authority to decide on what and how much food should be given, many therapists can't help effectively. The awareness for additional interactional problems influencing eating is left out by dieticians and SLPs, as they are not trained and may be anxious to be involved in psychological matters. It's wrong to suppose that it's only about the food. Thus, anybody feeling competent to give advice on ENS often just expresses his or her opinion, even if specialists would need to learn a lot before being educated and fit to help. Challenge one is the developmental stage of the child: infants and toddlers don't communicate verbally about their needs and pains but rather by symptoms and behavior. In this situation their parents function as their uncertified interpreters with the medical world.

Imbalances between expected intake and the amount of food some babies will manage may lead to additional problems between the baby and its caretakers due to unrealistic expectations of the feeding team. Slow progression either in the amount or joy of feeding may develop into a nightmare of ineffective or even stressful oral feeding. If counseling is ineffective and the feeding and intake deteriorates, it might lead to crisis. A mother's concern may quickly develop into stress, desperation, or even obsession with feeding and the well-being of the child. In 1996 we have already shown that mothers who were diagnosed with a variety of psychiatric illnesses (mainly depression) while their baby refused to eat (with or without ENS) recovered by 80% when they could feed their child again [2]. Feeding teams may not succeed if they are not aware of the pain, the worries, concerns, ambivalences, and sometimes desperation of parents. If they only take care of the psychological aspects of feeding interactions (as when families are referred to psychiatric institutions), this might lead to insufficient nutrition resulting in insufficient therapy for feeding issues.

An effective feeding team needs a high-level medical expertise to understand the details of the medical history of the problem and to be able to assess relevant physical aspects of the child in respect to peristaltic gut function, nutrition, or failure to thrive combined with differentiated know-how of confounding developmental or relationship-related issues. On the other hand, it also needs competence in addressing parents in a professional psychodynamic way, gently and with respect, but speaking frankly when in effective or even distressing parental feeding behaviors needs to change.

Tube maintenance, care, and aftercare are the responsibility of nutritionists, gastroenterologists, nurses, and other medical professionals. This is essential and indispensable. Details of any ENS must be adjusted individually and constantly according to body composition, age, underlying medical condition, severity of illness, and other issues like biorhythm, sleep preferences, and the child's tolerance to ENS. Second best is when the responsible follow-up team is composed of at least one experienced medical professional (authorized of making ENS-related decisions) and at least one paramedic (taking care of all related issues like feeding skills and individually tailored feeding plans). Including more professional perspectives could potentially be even better but also risks that too many professionals might bring too many perspectives to the table and the team may then not work sufficiently.

When counseling institutions in New Zealand, we found that the teams of SLPs and physiotherapists were very strong and many well trained also in this niche. One center in Christchurch was primarily designed to support children with Down syndrome. In the beginning, they needed mainly these two professions. When children became older and self-regulated, nutrition became an issue; family therapists and psychologists would also be integrated. To enlarge the team without a rising number of clients was financially unfeasible. With Mrs. Champion, we therefore decided to the train members of the existing team in the competences needed.

The theoretical origin of this model of "at least two professionals" composed of two explicitly different professions is based on research and literature on the "triadic concept" first published in the late 1980s and 1990s by Fivaz [3] and her group in Lausanne, CH. Their observation-based research followed and outgrew the concept of the classical "dyadic" attachment theory introduced by Bowlby [4] two decades earlier. The classical dyad was the mother-child couple, which was studied intensively first in monkeys and later on in humans in numerous studies. John Bowlby observed that the survival of the newly born is dependent on an "attachment system." This "system" induced the mother to protect her baby and made survival for it as well as physical and emotional stability possible. In the 1950s, Harry F. Harlow showed in monkey experiments [5] that a baby separated from its mother will seek for two goals: the monkey will cross the wall looking for a drinking bottle filled with milk and will then jump to a monkey-like figure composed of wire on which fur the bottle is fixed and a face depicted on a sheet of paper consisting of two eyes, a nose, and a mouth. The baby monkey will drink a sip from the bottle, hop to the artificial "mother," and vice versa. Sad enough these monkeys are like children placed into a foster home, when becoming adult monkey showed a distorted and reduced attachment to their infants, lose them while jumping from branch to branch, forget about them, etc. Harlow's experiments, which can't be reproduced these days because of animal protection plans, proved that attachment is essential to develop normal breeding behavior in primates.

John Bowlby [4] among others applied the findings of H. F. Harlow to *Homo sapiens sapiens*. He could show that in humans attachment happens instinctively and is essential for development. Without it, communication and speech development are delayed, and the outcome is less than preferable. The emotional competences like detecting feelings of other people, empathy, and the possibility of well-being in society request early attachment. Experiments like the "strange-situation test" by Mary Ainsworth [6] could demonstrate Bowlby's assumptions.

The triadic concept [7] of the Lausanne research group went one step further and included the third party, the father, into the scientific analysis of what matters for the child. The assumption, which was investigated and supported by impressive clinical experiments [8], was that any learning and development of young children happens in the context of "diverse but transparent options" represented by a "couple" constituted usually by the child's parents identifying and sometimes representing opposite topics and values separately, but in a joint social context. This includes issues like typically maternal versus paternal thoughts and plans. In everyday life, parents often see and interpret the world they live in with their child very differently. A simple task like bathing or feeding their child might already lead to discussions or even controversies. Parenting behavior will often occur after frequent discussions about issues of daily life with their infant. In any given situation, the child may choose reactions either leading to regression (withdrawing or showing fear, centripetal from the parent) or progression (diving forward into explorative behavior, centrifugal toward the parent). This may also be known as the decision between protection and exploration. The triadic concept offers the understanding of the "other side"—of a second, perhaps quite different opinion or perception of any given situation. The child profits and learns best, when both aspects are present or possibly contradictory options for various topics are offered by its parents. The infant will learn to differentiate that its mother is its mother, and she tends to be more protective than its father. Its father may be different; classically speaking he may be more responsible for exploration and learning new skills. The child learns that fathers and mothers are different individuals but form a couple, the result of which it owes its existence. The parents might have completely different opinions on a given specific subject, but both might be "well enough parents" as Winicott [9] names it. They will offer their child the knowledge that absolute truth doesn't exist; only different perspectives can be found and tested individually and in society.

Triadic communication is the experience of shared but diverse options offered by two people and seen and rated from the perspective of a third party: the child. Having said this, there is never ever a "right" or a "true" opinion, interpretation, or anything. There is no absolute truth; the best it gets is the perception and reflection of different perspectives and thus constructed conceptions of when and what is perceived as reality.

In the daily work of professionals in medical systems, each patient meets different people, often all at the same time but sometimes in different situations, and the perception of each person influences and changes the perception of the others. One classical situation would be medical rounds on a Monday morning done by a doctor in charge after a night shift and in a rush to get home. The doctor might enter the ward and be impatient to "get rid" of all patients who seem medically stable. He may recognize mainly the medical arguments and feel that his perspective is the right one and he is doing a good and responsible job based on his or her clinical experience. The nurse might be aware of additional social circumstances and oppose the doctor's decision. So sometimes a medically stable patient can't be discharged for various non-medical reasons. Psychosocial reasons, anxiety, or simply lack of a family or any other network which would be able to support the patient may hinder dismissal. The difference in perspectives needs to be discussed, and a decision could end up being a compromise. This could be called a "triadic solution." In this form, the doctor is like the father (progressive, putting the patient on the street), the nurse is like a phantomized mother (wants to comfort the patient, identifying with his or her anxieties and wants to support the patient by looking for other options), and the patient itself would be like "their child." The child feels the compassionate motherly impulses, while the father thrives to conquer the world. From this perspective, education should consist of two loving parents or primary caretakers (who of course to not need to be male and female) who have diverse tasks and thus different opinions regarding nearly every question. The child itself needs so much support that it is in a mental state desiring to learn. After 2000 this concept was adapted to a more modern/up-to-date new family concept. Now the "ideal" mother and father may be challenged with diverse social roles, while the inner concepts of parenthood have also changed. Nevertheless, progressive and supporting factors need to be present if education should lead to a self-confident child and adult.

Understanding and accepting the triadic concept theoretically as well as it's adaptation in a clinical environment is necessary for every team member. When cooperation requires the existence of different perspectives, proposals for decisions demand respect for each and every one. Especially traditionally powerful positions ask for humility. This is indispensable knowledge, which should lead to respect and equality, especially in professionals working with young and fragile children. On the joint awareness of respect and equality (within the group of the involved adults), learning becomes possible (for the child). Parents and professionals should be prepared to take new options into consideration. This learning attitude may offer the child during the shared time to make its own and maybe new and creative choice. The child may start eating with something unexpected or behave unexpectedly. Very little direct support is needed in this stage of new learning. In most of the cases, refraining from intervention, as well as parents and therapists acting as role models by eating, may be sufficient.

Refraining from education in table manners and choices of so-called healthy food may open up new doors for the timid children. To encourage new learning for all parties involved is necessary. Whether a parent or a therapist state that the child shows resistance is the same. Resistance arises only when learning by itself is obstructed. There may be too much "offering" of food or too restrictive interventions, or one can simply be pushing too hard. A balance between progressive and suitable factors is necessary, to prevent waste of time and emotional energy. If avoidant or even oppositional behavior is observed, the balance might be out of tune.

These kinds of behaviors are often results of force feeding, which has been unpleasant for the child. If the professional team may entangle in a struggle to feed the child against its will, this fight cannot be won because the child's closing lips, placing its tongue in front, and closing its pharyngeal cavity is much mightier than any parent can be. It may be necessary for the team of therapists to act in a triadic way, meaning that different approaches are seen as equal although they might be varied. This might stem from the different points of view of professionals due to their education. A SLP might want to try to change the sucking device, a physiotherapist offers to change the position of the child while being fed, and a psychotherapist might want to change the interaction in the family and perhaps parents' feelings. One or all approaches and ideas might be good and may lead to success. The triadic concept adds additional options: it allows one to confront parents with different approaches and let them and their child choose the way. We strongly advocate that teams should allow different views, approaches, and guidance. The research of Fivaz et al. provided us with the insight that parents should have different opinions, offering their child the opportunities of their different options.

Especially in critical situations when some team member will feel more worried or concerned than another about a symptom the child shows, the triadic concept allows a transparent analysis of the situation and more options from which the child will benefit. An interdisciplinary perspective will provide a multifaceted look and broaden the discussion, optimizing the balance between protective and challenging aspects during the process of tube weaning. ENS management and tube weaning will demand a trusting relationship between the feeding team and parents. Growth, functional, and nutritional parameters should be well explored before deciding on the best way to organize ENS for any infant or child. Experienced specialized professionals for tube-related guidance are crucial, and the lack of a responsible feeding team may harm the child and reduce its potential for oral rehabilitation.

Meeting with and observation of a tube-fed child in a "food-offering environment" means that food should be visible and available to the child without comments, intrusions, or feeding attempts; it should be attractive in looks, consistency, and smell and easily reachable for the child, if the capabilities due to age and special needs make it possible that the child helps itself. The analysis of typical eating situations at home (videos usually 1–2 min long) is another helpful piece of information for the feeding team. It allows the feeding team to get to know the child in its interaction with food and gain insight into its oral and tactile skills, as well as its motivation and attitude to food. It is possible to detect aversive and avoidant behavioral patterns which will make the following learning process difficult. Relevant questions are: Does the child touch food; will it lick, bite, or crush food in its mouth; is it likely to have taste sensations either by solid or liquid food? Additionally, how does the child move, how do parents, caretakers, siblings, or grandparents interact? Which educational standards and ideals do they practice, which feeding theories and methods seem to be an influence? If the child has special needs: how are they dealt with? In what position is the child during feeding: high chair, rocker, or is it fed while lying on its back? Does the child eat or drink by itself in a sitting position, standing up, and/or running around, or does he/she sit at the table as a part of the family being included in mealtime? Do other family members eat while the child eats, or is it being fed all alone? How does the child react, and what's the feeder's feedback?

The multidisciplinary feeding team should share the first impressions of the family, and a joint plan for transition to oral eating should be made. What goals do the child and his family want to achieve? What is realistic? Is the child medically stable and healthy enough to start with oral exploration, or are there physical restrictions? Can the child already touch and hold food by itself, can it sit in a stable position, can it understand and control its surroundings? What experiences have the parents undergone so far? What therapies have already been applied and have they been successful? What doubts and questions do parents have before weaning is started? Are they worried about weight loss? How much weight loss or gain can be tolerated? Who takes responsibility for medical decisions locally? How do the attending physicians at home feel about the transition to oral nutrition? Is the child on medication and which medication has an awful taste? Can and should the feeding team change or discontinue—after discussion with the physician in charge—the medication?

The specific topics concerning increasing or reducing the amount of tube feeds and the following weight loss are indispensable, but nevertheless create fears and anxieties within the team and parents. The two groups mirror each other's feelings. These feelings need to be handled with great care as denial will challenge the confidence. Adults who have experienced famine or might have been worried about a close relative suffering from self-induced famine as it may be in anorectic adolescents know how critical the issue of weight loss can become. Anxiety can easily induce an uncontrollable urge to feed the child, even if common sense and therapeutic guidance suggests waiting for the self-determined actions of the child. Tube-fed children mostly have never ever felt anything close to hunger. They live between phases of being comfortably full and saturated or being overfed and uncomfortably full or even nauseated and/or on the verge of vomiting. To allow 3 or more hours of no tube feeds is a welcome and probably pleasant change but will not lead to any kind of food-seeking behavior. Parents tried food restriction or even no tube feeds mostly lasting at most half a day, because they had little to no therapeutic support. This simply has not and will not work.

Another issue is that the sight of natural food nicely set on a table does not "communicate" with a tube-fed child the same way as it does with normally eating people. It does not "talk" to them. They see food the same way as one looks at a book or a piece of paper and does not dream of eating it, even if it has a nice color or smell! There is no link between food and the odor of food, which may lead to the urge to grab, want, or eat it. It takes some time after hunger, due to the reduction of tube feeds, for the child to feel uncomfortable and make the link between hunger, food, and eating it as a remedy. When preparing parents for the transition from ENT, the weight loss issue must be addressed and discussed. Unrealistic expectations like "My child will start to eat right away!" might otherwise harm the weaning project.

A tube-fed child does not know what to do with food. In children affected from food resistance but also in infant picky eaters, the child avoids any contact with food. They don't want to know what food is for. They know that parents would like them to eat properly, but they don't like food at all. It is sticky, smells awful, and takes valuable time in which they could have been playing or looking at an iPad or a movie. In the end one has to poop, which might be unpleasant as well. Don't underestimate the beliefs of a child's world. In the last years of life, the same might happen again: taste is often reduced to the cornerstones of salty, sweet, bitter, sour, and umami. One has eaten often enough, the lust for food is diminished, the ability to digest is reduced, and the whole process of preparing, chewing, swallowing, and digesting becomes strenuous. So old people start to reduce the variety of food and even refrain from eating. In the end they tend to become slim. The same is more or less true for infants; the whole process is arbitrary and awkward. Not being used to swallowing anything but one's own saliva, unknown taste or texture is rejected. The process of getting acquainted with the feeling of hunger and satiety, with smell and texture, will take time. No child will get food into its mouth before an intensive prior exploration has taken place; only then can the food be seen as safe and doesn't evoke anxiety. Parents serve in this process as role models as they may eat what the child could eat BUT without offering it to the infant or—even worse—trying to make the child eat. It's understandable that this behavior is counterintuitive as every parent wants to offer their child food. To serve "only" as role models, like a taster in a Sultan's home, who fears to be poisoned by the food served, is quite a challenge for parents.

Many tube-fed children are medically fragile patients who have often spent months in NICUs and are cautious and predisposed to anxiety. Anxiety has to be alleviated gradually. There may be other stressors on the child's side or in the family context, which occur during this first and delicate "getting to know the world of foods before thinking of actual swallowing" phase, which makes daily communication with the parents necessary. The Notube coaching team is therefore available 24/7/365 in 4–5 languages, and competence and availability help to build a sustainable trust relation.

We recommend all large tube placing institutions to establish an interdisciplinary feeding team with sufficient expertise to support each child and its family through the process of preparation for ENS, for tube management and subsequently the weaning process as well as aftercare. The specific task and role of all involved professions *during* the weaning process are described in a later chapter.

References

1. Justus von Liebig. Suppe für Saeuglinge – mit Nachtraegen in Beziehung auf ihre Bereitung und Anwendung. Braunschweig: Vieweg Verlag; 1866.
2. Dunitz-Scheer M, Scheer P, Trojovsky A, Kaschnitz W, Kvas E, Macari S. Changes in psychopathology of parents of NOFT (non-organic failure to thrive) infants during treatment. Eur Child Adolesc Psychiatry. 1996;5(2):93–100.
3. Elisabeth F-D, Antoinette C-W. Understanding triadic and family group interactions during infancy and toddlerhood. Clin Child Fam Psychol Rev. 1999;2(2):107–27.
4. Bowlby J. Attachment and loss: retrospect and prospect. Am J Orthopsychiatry. 1982;52(4):664–78. https://doi.org/10.1111/j.1939-0025.1982.tb01456.x. PMID: 7148988.
5. Harlow HF. The monkey as a psychological subject. Integr Psychol Behav Sci. 2008;42(4):336–47. https://doi.org/10.1007/s12124-008-9058-7. PMID: 18712577.
6. Bretherton I. Revisiting Mary Ainsworth's conceptualization and assessments of maternal sensitivity-insensitivity. Attach Hum Dev. 2013;15(5–6):460–84. https://doi.org/10.108 0/14616734.2013.835128. PMID: 24299130.
7. Han JH, Kim SA, Kim S, Park JY. Factors influencing disordered eating behavior based on the theory of triadic influence. Perspect Psychiatr Care. 2019;55(3):366–71. https://doi. org/10.1111/ppc.12308. Epub 2018 Jul 3. PMID: 29969148.
8. Simonelli A, Bighin M, de Palo F. Coparenting interactions observed by the prenatal Lausanne trilogue play: an Italian replication study. Infant Ment Health J. 2012;33(6):609–19. https://doi. org/10.1002/imhj.21350. Epub 2012 Aug 3. PMID: 28520113.
9. Grossmark R. Review of attachment, play, and authenticity: a Winnicott primer. Psychotherapy (Chic). 2009;46(4):498–9. https://doi.org/10.1037/a0017957. PMID: 22121847.

Medically fragile children (MFCs) with a non-progressive medical condition may require ENS for a specific period. Before tube placement, the expected duration of a temporary ENS to ensure growth and development should be well defined with distinct nutritional goals. These goals should include preparatory activities for future transition to oral intake like non-nutritive sucking or offering food to allow the child to smell it. In case of permanent tube placement, the main goal is to implement tube maintenance measures and prevent malnutrition. Additionally, a joint decision with parents should be made about the quality of food: formula feeding including all necessary nutrients, vitamins, etc. or self-made pureed food, which gives parents the feeling that they can contribute to the eating of their child. Dietary counseling is required to make sure that all necessary nutrients are included. We know parents whose desire to prepare all the food for their child was handled very badly. They were told that they are endangering their child's health and threatened by social services that they will keep a strict eye on them, eventually putting their child in foster care. We aren't in favor of such interactions between medical systems and parents. One should be convinced that both systems want the best for the child. None of the parties involved want to harm the child. Parents are knowledgeable because they love their child unconditionally. Medical personnel try to support the child and its parents but don't necessarily know better. Sometimes we even consider the extreme vomiting of children on permanent ENS because of parent's unwillingness or even disgust regarding industrialized food.

Oral skills, oral sensitivity, specific jaw motility, swallow function, suck and swallow coordination, possible taste preferences, chewing (in older children), and the general interest and motivation for food as well as hand-food motor coordination should be assessed before ENS is started. The knowledge of the child's abilities may form the maintenance program while on ENS and may influence possible oral activities during temporary ENS and lead to an earlier weaning of ENS.

Cognitive, emotional, and sensory development of children should be diagnosed before and monitored during ENS. Early diagnosis of developmental disorders is

55
M. Dunitz-Scheer, P. J. Scheer, *Child-led Tube-management and Tube-weaning*,
https://doi.org/10.1007/978-3-031-09090-5_6

necessary because early treatment is required. Impairment of sensory perception or other developmental disorders (like autistic spectrum disorders—ASD) influence the effect of ENS and the consecutive weaning process.

As some severely impaired infants have potential for unforeseen recovery, a statement like "nil by mouth" because of fear from aspiration or signs of aspiration on VFSS deserves re-evaluation in all cases of non-progressive health impairment at least every 6 months. Re-evaluation is in any case compulsory when the child's mental, sensory, and motor development shows a positive tendency. We feel that this sentiment, which appears to be a diagnosis, is in reality a condemnation. Children who want to eat and seem to be able to do so and can swallow their saliva aren't even allowed to lick or to try food. Parents are held responsible for keeping their child away from food and following the strict ENS regime. But MDs seem to forget that every reflux and even more every vomiting brings liquid into the esophagus or the mouth, which must be processed. If a child aspirates food, it will do so as a sequela of reflux as well. We remember a 6-month-old child from Poland who had been to The Hospital for Sick Children at Great Ormond Street, London, a high-class British hospital. The spell of "nil-by-mouth" was laid on Nadja, a severely handicapped child, which was fed on its mother's lap both looking in the same direction. The mother couldn't see her child's face. Mother and child had no eye contact and mother couldn't detect any nonverbal signs of hunger or longing or withdrawal from Nadja. She was coughing frequently during feeding and spitting a lot. When being placed in a stable upright position on a cushion facing her mother, feeding began. Maria could interact with her child now. We taught her to detect more and more of Nadja's cues and facial expressions. Maria and her child became entangled in a fruitful interaction and to her mother's sheer delight, Nadja finally learned to eat. The hard facts, which would have pointed to recurrent aspiration as in pneumonias or at least bronchitis showing a typical X-ray, didn't exist in Nadja's case. Being aware that aspiration is dangerous in MFCs, we nevertheless are questioning the "nil-by-mouth" condemnation.

Important information, which should be considered and shared with parents before tube placement are the nutritional goals, i.e., benefits but also drawbacks to tube feeding. To know as much as possible about ENS empowers parents to make a joint decision with professionals. Tube placement should be decided consensually. Parents need to be aware of the dis-/advantages of nutritional treatment by tube. They should be able to understand the expected effects and desired outcome of ENS. Most feeding tubes are fitted in children who are too young to even understand. But if a toddler or an older child can understand it, then it should be addressed by professionals. Consent can only be given by somebody who understands the consequences and risks of the intended treatment or its absence. It needs intellectual capacity and emotional openness to be able to consent. ENS can be explained only to parents starting from a point of emotional openness and the ability to listen given at a specific moment. If parents fear for the survival of their child, they may be so distracted that they give consent without thinking. This may also be true when parents have never been in a NICU and try to cope with the unexpected lifesaving measures for their child, which is in the mother's subconscious still in her womb happy and satiated. If possible, consent should be attained after adaptation of not only the child in the new environment but also of the parents.

Most children start ENS by an NG tube. The NG tube is less invasive, but the tube needs to be changed on a regular basis. It can cause irritation of the nose and throat and requires tapering onto the cheeks; something that is not only uncomfortable but it's also highly visible. Every other person on the street might comment on it, which is extremely unpleasant for parents as they feel inadequate not being able to feed their own child. An NG tube should be used in temporary ENS, because either the period of treatment is planned for a short duration or ENS is an additional therapy needed, for example, while the child requires oxygen support.

The placement of PEG and/or JPEG tubes will require a general anesthesia bearing the risks of it. Depending on the underlying medical condition and any other procedures being performed at the same time, the PEG or JPEG is inserted in nearly all cases by endoscopy. Children adapt to tube feeding diversely. We find that the earlier in life they receive a tube, the easier they adapt. However, it also depends on the child's development, personality, general health, support, and parent's willingness. Some parents are afraid of delivering food using a pump: they want to feed their child by themselves using bolus therapy. It may very well be that a given child copes better with ENS that way, but denial of pump-feeding may be more often a psychological denial than a rational decision based on observations. Parents waking up using an alarm clock to feed their child with a syringe remind us of mothers nursing their child whenever breast milk is needed. Some children cope better when night feeds are applied; some can't have that at all. In every case, decisions are only partly rational, and the emotional part has to be respected. Making fun of or telling parents that they are wrong doesn't help. Additionally medical personnel have their own emotions, which may be presented as rational decisions but aren't.

Being involved in the decision to tube-feed one's child is stressful for parents. The idea of not being able to feed one's child can provoke feelings of shame and depression and may even be intimidating for parents. In a planned tube placement, parents can be advised to seek information from professionals, friends, and online forums. Some of these can be excellent sources of information, while others may offer a highly biased view based on experiences and opinions from other parents. What can be helpful for one family might be harmful to another. The idea of any invasive procedure being done to one's own child is frightening. Tube placement is intrusive and imposes a heavy burden of responsibility on parents later. In most cases, a good relationship between the medical team and the family is helpful to make sure that the parents have been made fully aware of the indication for tube feeding, have learned a lot about side effects, and have been given the time to ask questions.

If the child's diagnosis requires permanent tube feeding, such as in severe neuromuscular illnesses or metabolic disorders requiring a highly specific nutrient intake, the medical team's recommendation and decision to place a tube may come as a relief to parents.

But when tube feeding is intended as a temporary support, for example, to feed a child prior to surgery or as part of the therapy in a NICU, in both cases it is extremely important to define goals for the tube feeding. These goals should be defined in terms of nutrition and growth. Medical professionals rely on tube feeding because it provides essential nutritional support for their young and fragile patients during difficult times. But the decision to start tube feeding should not be taken lightly and demands consideration of the specific situation of each child, as well as the team's clinical experience, the use of medical guidelines, as well as the consent of the parents unless it is done in an emergency. Bearing in mind that children are not only energy-consuming systems, but sensitive individuals, expectations based on published data and general medical consent may not apply to a specific child. So mostly the decision to start tube feeding is based on the likelihood that without it, the child won't survive or at least not thrive. Undoubtedly, tube feeding is essential and lifesaving, but in medicine situations aren't always clear cut. Diverse opinions between different sub-specialists, therapists, and the nursing staff may arise. Therefore, we recommend (whenever possible) to make the decision among the team before involving parents. Otherwise, confusion or even loss of confidence is risked. We do write this knowing that most colleagues follow these guidelines correctly. On the other hand, parents have told us that they felt overwhelmed by the situation of a preterm delivery, seeing their child in an incubator supported by a lot of tubes and monitor devices, while being asked for consent for tube placement. Additionally, they didn't know what to expect and had no idea that their child might be discharged while still on ENS. It might take more than one interaction with parents and may need time without the child in a separate room with the member of the team in charge of the decision for ongoing ENS to reach mutual understanding. We don't recommend sending, for example, a dietician—equipped with all forms of consent—to an interaction with parents in which this team member can offer only one option because the *pouvoir* is limited. Josef, a 3-year-old infant who endured 3 near-miss events during his NICU stay, was a notable case. Parents were called in during nights to say goodbye to Josef. The decision to feed him by ENS was never questioned. Tube placement was part of the program after resuscitation. Josef survived, thrived, and as dismissal was imminent; parents were trained in tube feeding and eventually replacement. It seemed natural and a little shade on Josef after his life had been saved. Learning that the ENS was no longer necessary, parents sought help for transition to oral eating. Trying to revisit the scene in which they had been asked for consent to ENS, they couldn't make one appear. Finding out that no one within the NICU team felt responsible for tube weaning, they applied for a treatment in the Notube Eating-School.

When we were still working in the hospital, we trained the staff of the NICU to be able to talk about ENS and its termination with parents. The main change we introduced was that ENS was from then on an important part of competence for all professionals, especially before a child was dismissed.

It is necessary to ensure that a team specializes in support and care for tube-fed children in aftercare. They should optimize the treatment and manage nutritional, developmental, and growth issues by monitoring and eventually changing feeding amounts. Good maintenance, aftercare, and access to options for diverse programs for the transition to oral eating should be offered.

The decision to start tube feeding is highly significant. Our key message is to make sure that the medical team is able to find a joint decision, which can be shared with the parents to ensure consensus in all situations possible. The idea is that this is the best treatment option and that there are plans and targets in place. Eventually the termination of tube feeding in the future should be included and communicated.

Professionals interested in ENS and specifically temporary ENS and tube weaning might be questioned as to their experience and view regarding the timing of weaning in clear cases of temporary intention. Historically we answered this question according to the knowledge of our physiotherapist Eva Kerschischnik. The assumption is that a child should be able to sit on its own to make swallowing possible. Nowadays we answer the question more differently, if a child does not aspirate and can swallow its own saliva and shows even little hunger signs it can be weaned. We have already weaned infants suffering from severe cerebral palsy after being a preterm baby who couldn't see or hear and had nearly no muscular tone. They couldn't sit, and some of them will never be able to do so. In the end, we became much braver and started to wean children who in the end will be able to enjoy eating as one of their main with the world.

Every feeding team should have an opinion on whether a child should be fed permanently by ENS. For some children, permanent ENS has a lot of benefits and advantages. Children showing signs of dysphagia, e.g., recurrent coughing, inability of swallowing, and necessity to feed them for an hour at each time, could be better off when being fed by ENS. Having said that, we remember children being kept on ENS who showed side effects, especially signs of overfeeding like retching and vomiting so intensely that ENS was a disadvantage. Furthermore, we had families in which the psychosocial burden of ENS was enormous, as nobody felt competent to look after the tube or change the drip, the family couldn't go on trips, parents couldn't go out for dinner, and even attending school events with the siblings of the affected child was impossible. In one of our Eating-Schools, we treated a 9-month-old infant suffering from the results of preterm delivery as described. She was the last child of three, her mother being a veterinarian in Saskatchewan, Canada. The whole family, which had been very well organized having three children and both parents at work, was immobilized due to the ENS of little Chiara. Side effects of ENS led to 10–15 times/day vomiting. The feeding, refeeding, and cleaning took all the spare hours of her parents. We gave it a try. Chiara loved eating by herself after

© The Author(s), under exclusive license to Springer Nature
Switzerland AG 2022
M. Dunitz-Scheer, P. J. Scheer, *Child-led Tube-management and Tube-weaning*,
https://doi.org/10.1007/978-3-031-09090-5_7

we reduced the ENS feeds dramatically. She longed for more; partly she didn't swallow but dropped pureed food out of her mouth. In the beginning, feeding took a long time but still less than the procedure before. The smell was much better as Chiara stopped vomiting, and the best was that everybody could feed Chiara. The family functions recovered as did our colleague Martha who had felt helpless seeing Chiara vomiting nearly all day.

When degenerative progression of (neurological) illnesses is expected, staying on ENS can be very helpful. On the other hand, eating might be one of the few exchanges with the world and a source of joy and happiness. Even children being born with genetic errors like trisomy 18 might benefit from eating. Lifespan is short and not influenced by the way the child is fed. Being able to feed the child orally allows parents to entangle in a loving interaction with their child who may be a present but can't stay. Years later, we got letters from these parents who remember a happy first year with their severely handicapped child. It's always the same question, which goal are we seeking when prescribing ENS? If it's only the adequacy of nutrition according to percentiles, then the attempt to deliver sufficient nutrition should be re-evaluated looking through the eyes of the child and its parents. If the child feels better being fed by ENS, an attempt to wean it shouldn't be due to the parent's wishes alone.

In children suffering from metabolic disorders with the need of ingesting very badly tasting formulas (like phenylketonuria or on a ketogenic diet), ENS might be better. Nevertheless, children might adapt to the bad taste like we see in children dependent on amino acids alone because they lack the ability to split up protein. The formula called Neocate or Peptisorb smells and tastes badly, it is given in the first month, and it may very well be that the child adapts as adults do when exposed to a low-salt diet due to hypertension or kidney failure. We tend to try even in these children to feed them orally. Sometimes the exact amount of protein or fatty acids needs to be calculated. For these cases, we undertook extensive interactions with colleagues from the metabolic department while still working in hospital. Stefan was sent to us suffering from an inborn error of metabolism for the sake of tube weaning. First day of his inpatient stay, the doctor from the metabolic department came together with a dietician and prescribed the food. Both ladies didn't leave the ward without saying that this prescription must be followed; otherwise we could be held responsible for threatening the child's life. They wanted to shock us, and they did. Especially our nurses, including the head nurse of the ward, were anxious to get the child to eat. Weight loss after reducing the quantity or quality of food was out of question. We started to work on interaction and set up a group of people fighting against their anxiety induced by harsh doctors by sticking to guidelines. We were a bunch of anxious people knowing that even when we all followed all the rules, the death of the child was imminent and his lifespan limited. Reflection on our anxiety as well as institutional problems like "why has the child been sent to our ward instead to the competent metabolic department?" helped us and in the end helped the child and its family as well. In the end, the child ate the required amount of amino acids orally after all of us had overcome the perceived threat.

The argument of easier hygienic control in cases of immunological depressed children by applying ENS is wrong. A PEG is always a hole through the skin into the bowels. Skin irritations and wild flesh are common complications in healthy children. Superinfections of the skin surrounding the introitus are common. Hygiene is tricky because the acidic liquid from the stomach irritates the skin in of itself. Additionally, the child may play with its PEG and scratch and deliver even stool germs into the already irritated skin. The calculability of calories ingested is one of the main arguments for permanent ENS. To calculate calories is in our eyes a myth. Children don't ingest all calories prescribed or, as already stated a couple of times, vomit it partly or totally. Additionally, a child is not a machine. For example, feeding during nighttime without any control over the calories ingested might lead to a less efficient digestion, meaning that the uptake of calories might be smaller than expected. We do see children being fed according to very well-prepared diet plans who don't thrive or are even malnourished. The reason in the end is unknown. To suppose that a child doesn't digest as well when being fed during its sleep is not proven. It's an assumption as it's an assumption that sufficient calories given lead directly to thriving.

This chapter will therefore deal with the issue of when and how to decide if enteral feeding will be a transient feeding technique for a few weeks or months to overcome critical phases or clear-cut medical interventions like surgical operations, an organ transplant, or even chemotherapy. The other option is that a tube will become part of a permanent enteral feeding regime of a chronically sick (e.g., kidney insufficiency) or severely disabled (e.g., severe cerebral palsy including dysphagia) or prolonged fragile medical state (e.g., awaiting final surgery, be it cardiac, gastrointestinal, or other) child. It may be obvious that parents should be informed as early as possible when the medical team is discussing the necessity for tube placement. Parents should be involved in the decision-making unless it happens during resuscitation. This recommendation is made to ease parents' resistance when ENS deprives them of their feeding interaction. Not being able to feed one's own child in a natural way could have a massive psychological impact on parents and their emotional readiness to accept the decision for ENS as being beneficial for their child.

For short-term tube feeding (4–12 weeks), a small diameter NG tube should be chosen. The European Society of Pediatric Gastroenterology and Nutrition (ESPHGAN) suggests fine-bore tubes (silicon or polyurethane) over polyvinylchloride tubes as these can be left in place for up to 8 weeks and are often softer and easier to place. Potential problems like limited tolerance of thickened food, blockage, misplacement, or unintended removal still remain. Tube blockage can develop, for example, due to crushed medication, missed flushing, or protein precipitation. Tubes should be therefore flushed regularly before and after use with 5–10 ml of water.

Children with chronic conditions may be more prone to self-induced tube dislodgement triggered by nasopharyngeal discomfort associated with or without sore throat, dry mucous membranes, reduced saliva production, and dysphagia. In children with an impaired gag reflex, accidental endobronchial placement of nasogastric tubes can occur with subsequent perfusion of enteral formulas into the lung. To prevent this, the position of the tube must be checked after each placement and before each feeding. This sounds easier than it is; for years we used litmus paper to prove that the aspirate from the tube is acidic. This isn't done any more. Simple observation of the aspirate or looking at the child whether it is coughing may be insufficient in handicapped children. In the end permanent surveillance is the only recommended measure when feeding a child via tube. Visceral perforations of the esophagus and trachea, rarely a thorax containing the nutrition, or a pneumothorax happen. To avoid all that, gentle insertion is necessary.

Almost every NG tube-fed child suffers from gastroesophageal reflux due to some factors like overfeeding or the tube inhibits full closing of the cardia (by the midriff). For an intended tube feeding period of longer than 2–3 months, the tube recommended is a PEG feeding tube, which lies in the stomach or is placed into the jejunum. Placement of a PEG has no advantage other than it doesn't irritate the nose and therefore breathing. Gastroesophageal reflux disease (GERD) could be improved or worsened due to overfeeding. Antacid medication may be helpful to prevent heartburn and in the end Barret's disease. But reduction of acid in the stomach may reduce appetite, and there is evidence that proton-pump inhibitors (PPIs) enhance the number of intestinal allergies because allergens from the nutrition reach lower parts of the intestinal system. Additionally, prokinetic medication is administered in some countries. It rarely helps and might be dangerous in MFCs because it may lead to neurogenic ileus.

Administering a PEG tube is often recommended when an NG tube causes reflux. But GERD may be a result of the amount of food given and the inability of the child to control the amount or prepare for ingestion both mentally and endocrinologically (by releasing cerebral and intestinal neurotransmitters). The change of the tube is not an adequate cure. It is necessary—if possible—to teach the child to eat and reduce amounts right away, sometimes against current guidelines. Vomiting is one of the most aversive experiences after eating and reduces the lust for food tremendously. Reducing reflux and/or vomiting is the first step of learning to eat. A gastric PEG is better than a jejunal as it allows bolus feeding, resulting in more physiological enzyme activation and enteral hormone profile and greater time intervals in which the child is free from the tube feeds. Jejunal feeding should be restricted to children with tube-related aspirations, intractable gastroesophageal reflux, or any other medical condition that requires bypassing the stomach.

7.1　Typical Criteria for Primary Decision of Nasogastric Tube Placement

1. Extreme prematurity, to be weaned before primary discharge from NICU.
2. Unclear, diagnostically not yet specified dysphagia.
3. Duration of ENT is expected to be less than 2 months.
4. A short-term inability to meet nutritional requirements.
5. Oral aversion due to acute infections of the mouth, throat, or esophagus.

6. GERD if associated with failure to thrive (FTT).
7. Failure to thrive of unknown origin (not of metabolic or illness).
8. Infantile anorexia with acute malnutrition.

7.2   Typical Criteria for Primary Decision for a G(astric)-Tube PEG or J(ejunal)PEG Feeding Tube

1. Impossibility of nasogastric passage due to anatomical anomalies (choanal atresia, esophageal membrane, gastroschisis, omphalocele, etc.)
2. Dysphagia of neurological origin.
3. Facial anomalies requiring primary surgery.
4. Cleft palate, cheilognathopalatoschisis.
5. Esophageal atresia.
6. Duodenal and/or anal atresia.
7. CDH: congenital diaphragmatic hernia.
8. Complex cardiac anomalies requiring multiple surgeries.
9. Any severe, progressive, and complex medical situation, which is not expected to be solved within 2–3 months.

The choice between temporary and permanent enteral feeding should be made as early as possible. Even on ENS, a child may fail to thrive or become malnourished when vomiting reduces ingestion dramatically. Before administering a tube, all early feeding problems and/or interactive conflicts should be ruled out. This is done by psychological counseling in preparation for ENT. In case of permanent ENT, early indication enables the child and its family to adjust to that situation for which stable maintenance structures are needed.

Assessment and Stimulation of Oral Skills *during* ENT

The key to understanding early eating and drinking development as well as its disturbances remains the careful observation of repeated feeding sequences. They demonstrate the range of effective as well as ineffective behaviors of the tube-fed child. Observable dysfunctional eating patterns offer useful hints of sensory issues and show discrete neurological problems. They may also indicate emotional conflicts and eventually the psychological origin of avoidant behavior of the preverbal child. Avoidance may have felt necessary earlier on, for example, when the child didn't like oral interventions during intensive care. The intention of the medical interventions was good and not at all meant harmfully, but the child was subjected to every intervention like a victim for weeks or even months. It experienced the interventions as a threat. By intruding into the oral cavity, medical personnel transgressed an intimate border of oral autonomy.

The knowledge of influences on enteral feeding as well as about previous medical actions like tube placement and its impact on physical and emotional development may help professionals. A nonintrusive and "child-led" approach could be applied when dealing with the child being watchful of its cues and reactions. Especially in MFCs, nonverbal cues might be weak and not easy to recognize. Nevertheless, to observe and interpret them correctly is a prerequisite for transition to oral feeding. We learnt from parents that they encountered a habit of medical personnel commenting negatively toward inappropriate or dysfunctional feeding and eating behavior of infants, sometimes labeling parents with a psychiatric diagnosis. In this context, we address the "labeling" discussion in psychiatry as a method of how to "make somebody ill" by giving a diagnosis. Marguerite Dunitz et al. [1] could show in extensive research 1996 that the "psychiatric diagnosis" is in an exacerbated form in mothers after their child learned to eat. To be unable to sustains one's child sufficiently leads to severe disturbances and may appear like a disorder.

To label parents using a psychiatric diagnosis doesn't establish a trustworthy relationship and doesn't solve the child's problem. It pushes medically traumatized infants receiving ENT as well as their families into the field of psychiatry, in the

M. Dunitz-Scheer, P. J. Scheer, *Child-led Tube-management and Tube-weaning*, https://doi.org/10.1007/978-3-031-09090-5_8

hands of professionals who aren't trained and mostly not interested in ENS and tend to avoid the pediatric issues involved. New contenders enter the battleground of ENS feeling responsible for counseling disturbed parents, while the arousal is caused only by the anxiety and sorrows regarding the child's rearing. Misunderstandings and bad feelings of parents because they feel transported into psychiatry challenge the relationship with the feeding team. In the end parents may become more and more angry, and the pediatric staff may feel more and more incompetent to handle the situation. The solution seems simple re-evaluation of the therapeutic approach based on respect toward the child and its parents.

We remember Franz, a 3-year-old who was born prematurely in the 23rd week of pregnancy weighing 465 grams, having suffered from intrauterine growth retardation (IUGR) due to placenta insufficiency. Catch-up growth can't be expected if IUGR takes place before the 24th week of gestation. Nevertheless, feeding was prescribed intending that Franz would catch up and get into the normal percentile range. Parents tried hard to follow the prescription but failed. Franz refused the amount of ENT, and if parents gave it although he was retching, he vomited. When addressing the feeding team with their problem, it didn't change the prescription. Emotions on both sides got out of control, and parents were transferred to psychiatric counseling. Parents refused this referral and came to our clinic. Relieving the family from the spell of "catch-up" opened a new door for fruitful interaction and helped Franz to learn to eat. Surprisingly he enhanced his weight orally easier after a 3-month period of standstill.

At the beginning, the child itself must be seen, observed, and examined either on-site or on videos. An analysis of interactions between medical institutions and families should be done since intrusive, delayed, or—in worst case—ineffective nutritional support might have led to a deterioration of the feeding problem and increased parental stress. It may be a wrong idea of institutions to transfer children on ENT to "psycho-departments" for the sole sake of time and expertise for desperate parents assuming that the personnel in another department will be willing to offer. Psychologists and psychiatrists normally have no training in enteral feeding or experience with children suffering from chronic diseases. Transfer may waste only time and lead to frustration on all sides.

The Notube team's perspective of taking care of children on ENS consists of several steps: in the following section, we are going to outline the essential steps of assessment, maintenance, and tube weaning in such a way that experts can understand our process. At Notube, we predominantly meet children because they haven't learnt to eat. At the time, when general development in healthy infants makes learning to eat functionally possible, these infants may have been too weak or too sick to start eating. We assume that there exists a "sensitive slot" for learning to drink and eat (Birch LL et al. [2] gives in her review a hint in that direction but mostly scientific papers address the food itself and the way it's fed and not the time when eating is learned). This slot was not utilized when the child was able and interested in oral feeds or missed for any reasons, be it surgical interventions or a transient disease, which made learning to eat at that time impossible. Any birth situation needing to integrate the unexpected situation of a newly born infant not able or not allowed to be fed will not be easy. It will cause stress, fears, insecurity, and pressurizing expectations in the involved adults, and these emotions may affect the child. The mouths of MFCs are often not used at all for eating for many months resulting in it being unresponsive, defensive, or aversive against food. If this happens, one can observe that even the sight or the most subtle approach of food will lead to turning of the head away or retching or the child pushing itself away if physically possible or—if not—crying: "I don't want!". One must learn to understand that expressing a clear nonverbal cue telling "No!" or any refusing cue or behavior is always a positive. It's an expression of the already developed child's will. Why the will develops before conscience and understanding is unknown. It might be more important to want something or decisive not than to understand it. When a child can express a "No," it will be able to say "Yes" as well. Therapists can't overrule a child's will but must respect its urges. By doing so a trustworthy relation may evolve. A good and strong "No!" is much more promising than no reaction at all and may help to find the first gentle moves toward change. Furthermore, many of these children are orally hypersensitive after having experienced oral traumatization and painful oral manipulations in their early childhood such as suction of their saliva by pump or re-intubation making them overly sensitive to any direct stimulation. French authors [3] suspected that the lack of positive oral stimulation leads to a progression of the gagging reflex, being released already when the lips are touched. They call this development an "antecedent" of the gagging reflex, which is normally only triggered by pieces of food at the velum palatinum or at the uvula when a crumb or liquid tends to then take the false route and may be aspirated.

Some children receive feeding tubes in the first year of life, merely because their growth is unsatisfactory. But it may be that children who were too small already during early pregnancy (early IUGR—before the 24th week) take longer to catch up [4] as mentioned before. Catch-up growth may be expected in these children if they receive an aggressive nutritional support [5]. Others may suffer from reflux (GERD) [6] resulting in heartburn. All that may lead to the insertion of a feeding tube and subsequently causing one to miss the timeslot in which learning to eat is possible. When eating doesn't start at all, the staff will be grateful that tube feeding is possible. But if the tube is used longer than necessary, the child and its caretakers might miss the moment when it could learn to eat by itself. In counseling parents of former preemies, we need to find out whether their children have ever eaten anything by mouth. When assessing the child using video analysis, we decide about the child's potential to learn to eat by looking at the child's reaction to fluid and to food. We see whether it avoids it, whether the child is fed and eats or withdraws, and whether the child has no hunger because it received ENT just before. We would like to know if the child is satiated; whether it's able to be positioned according to its age for feeding; and whether feeding follows the child's needs or parents' wishes. Assessment should respect warnings in doctor's letters stating that eating could be dangerous for the child due to clinical assumption or a test, which indicates aspiration or that the eating might be too stressful for a very frail child. All this information will be considered in the assessment, and a child once found suitable for tube weaning is one who we believe will be able learn to eat and enjoy it. The assessment is an essential starting point of our tube weaning program.

To ensure an adequate assessment and estimation of suitability for the goal of transitioning from ENS to oral intake, some essential child-specific information needs to be collected in advance. For the sake of gathering the biometric, medical, nutritional, developmental, and tube-relevant data of the child, we use an online parent questionnaire designed and validated by the Notube team. It is also possible to use a collection of questions selected by any feeding center or institution. All medical reports from hospital stays be it immediately after birth or later, any other relevant medical reports of the child, as well as—if there was a very long inpatient history—a summary from the viewpoint of the parents should be compiled. It might be the case that medical reports are written in a foreign language not accessible to the team. In such cases, parents should be required to have the important reports translated into English. It is crucial to know whether a child can swallow safely and how safe swallowing is. This sounds easier than it is: the tests used by ENT doctors, like VFSS, may be false positive because the child was unsettled and cried while the test was done [7, 8]. Swallow studies made for the sake of out ruling "silent aspiration" using X-ray may be false positive [9] because the child was not hungry while the study was done or the viscosity of the test meal was inadequate for the child. There are new tests (like the so-called cookie test used in the Children's Hospital of Pittsburgh [10]) using parent's support of the child and cookies instead of bad-tasting liquids of different viscosity.

Asking about the anamnesis, i.e., whether the child suffered from recurrent pneumonias or coughs a lot after an oral intake, may be even more informative as the sometimes uncertain results of technically difficult tests, which need the cooperation of the infant. The term "silent aspiration [11]" might be helpful to describe situations where a severely handicapped child gets fluid or even nutrition into the trachea due to an inadequate swallowing or due to an inability to recognize that the fluid took a wrong way [12]. Nevertheless, it seems to us that in our clientele, the term is more often used than appropriate. To assess the safety of swallowing, it might be helpful for a feeding team to cooperate with an experienced ENT or a SLP while being in the diagnostic process. Invasive examinations should be carefully discussed before as their results may define the ability to learn to eat. Only when performed by experienced professionals and in a calm and cooperative performance of the child itself they are of value. We question the results of Velayutham et al. [12] because this was a retrospective study and didn't respect the situation of parents, children, and researchers as they weren't documented.

In addition, all significant information on the underlying main diagnoses as well past surgeries or any invasive and/or consuming treatment must be collected as well as medical interventions that might be planned soon. Developmental and neurological assessment and basic blood tests and relevant test results by other specialists should be collected. Only based on a full and complete summary of a medically fragile patient's former history and current state a valid assessment of suitability can be met. Ultimately the decision will be possible whether the referred child is ready for transition from enteral to exclusive oral feeding.

References

1. Duniz M, Scheer PJ, Trojovsky A, Kaschnitz W, Kvas E, Macari S. Changes in psychopathology of parents of NOFT (non-organic failure to thrive) infants during treatment. Eur Child Adolesc Psychiatry. 1996;5(2):93–100. https://doi.org/10.1007/BF01989501. PMID: 8814415
2. Birch LL, Doub AE. Learning to eat: birth to age 2 y. Am J Clin Nutr. 2014;99(3):723S–8S. https://doi.org/10.3945/ajcn.113.069047. Epub 2014 Jan 22. PMID: 24452235
3. Cascales T, Olives J-P. « Tu vas manger! » Trouble alimentaire du nourrisson et du jeune enfant : du refus au forçage alimentaire. Spirale. 2012/2;62:26–34.
4. Young A, Andrews ET, Ashton JJ, Pearson F, Beattie RM, Johnson MJ. 'Catch-up' growth of infants with IUGR does not significantly contribute to the whole-cohort weight gain pattern. Arch Dis Child Fetal Neonatal Ed. 2019;104(6):F663–4. https://doi.org/10.1136/archdischild-2019-317566. Epub 2019 Jul 30. PMID: 31362940
5. Hack M, Schluchter M, Cartar L, Rahman M, Cuttler L, Borawski E. Growth of very low birth weight infants to age 20 years. Pediatrics. 2003;112:1.
6. Gulati IK, Jadcherla SR. Gastroesophageal reflux disease in the neonatal intensive care unit infant: who needs to be treated and what approach is beneficial? Pediatr Clin N Am. 2019;66(2):461–73. https://doi.org/10.1016/j.pcl.2018.12.012. Epub 2019 Feb 1. PMID: 30819348; PMCID: PMC6400306
7. McNair J, Reilly S. The pros and cons of videofluoroscopic assessment of swallowing in children. 2003. In: Database of abstracts of reviews of effects (DARE): quality-assessed reviews [internet]. York: Centre for Reviews and Dissemination (UK); 1995. https://www.ncbi.nlm.nih.gov/books/NBK69701. Seen on 12/27/2018.
8. Coon ER, Srivastava R, Stoddard GJ, Reilly S, Maloney CG, Bratton SL. Infant videofluoroscopic swallow study testing, swallowing interventions, and future acute respiratory illness. Hosp Pediatr. 2016;6:12.
9. Shay EO, Meleca JB, Anne S, Hopkins B. Natural history of silent aspiration on modified barium swallow studies in the pediatric population. Int J Pediatr Otorhinolaryngol. 2019;125:116–21. https://doi.org/10.1016/j.ijporl.2019.06.035. Epub 2019 Jul 2. PMID: 31295702
10. http://www.chp.edu/our-services/radiology/patient-procedures/modified-barium-swallow. Seen on 12/27/2018.
11. https://www.cedars-sinai.org/health-library/diseases-and-conditions%2D%2D-pediatrics/a/aspiration-in-babies-and-children.html. This explantation was seen on 12/27/2018.
12. Velayutham P, Irace AL, Kawai K, Dodrill P, Perez J, Londahl M, Mundy L, Dombrowski ND, Rahbar R. Silent aspiration: who is at risk? Laryngoscope. 2018;128(8):1952–7. https://doi.org/10.1002/lary.27070. Epub 2017 Dec 27. PMID: 29280496

Although the composition of modern formulas is calculated perfectly according to the daily nutritional needs of the infant, the volume tolerance of ENS might be an issue for sensitive children. Individual volume tolerances vary depending heavily on the age, gastric size, personality, and different hunger-satiety biorhythms of the child. In the end even local customs may play a role: whereas in Europe and the USA industrialized formula is advocated, other regions like India and Southeast Asia prefer home-cooked blended food. Individually tailored feeding schedules and smaller volumes may be favorable. We advise to coordinate tube feeds with every-day meal schedules and other social norms like day nursery to encourage the child's participation in "normal" meals. This is to facilitate engagement in food-related activities as well as tactile, smell, and taste stimulation. In children with JPEG, continuous feeding should be adjusted to the child's social routine offering at least 1–2 periods of 2–3 h without being connected to the tube.

Regarding caloric contents of formulas and food supplements (as in Quigely et al., 2018 [1] and many others), we would like to propose that the "clinical" impression at "first glance" of a child's state of health, development, and growth by an experienced observer serves in most cases as a good enough estimation of the nutritional status. Young children will and must grow, but most children do not grow linearly. Growth is determined by epigenetic influences as well as intake, consumption, and metabolism leading to phases of weight gain and/or growth. Short-term illness might decrease a child's intake dramatically leading to less or stagnating weight gain for days or weeks. The weight curve of toddlers is more akin to a stair-case than a line. Parents confronted with insufficient weight gain by medical personnel will become stressed, exposing the child to increased expectations and pressure which rarely increases its appetite and intake. Assessments should not only document weight, length, and head circumference but also listen to parent's report on their child's appetite, favorite food, and average daily intake before prescribing clinical tests. To assess the nutritional status, it is essential to use growth charts [2] to follow the trend of length, weight, and head circumference. Total daily supply should be calculated based on weight-for-age only up to the age of 2 years. Medically fragile children with an ongoing requirement of hospitalization cannot be expected to grow age appropriately. Therefore, after 2 years, volume calculation should be based on weight-for-height. Energy requirement is calculated according to weight-for-age and length-for-age for children under 2 years as stated in the DACH an acronym for Germany, Austria, and Switzerland) reference values [3]. Increased caloric needs in certain diagnostic groups, including inborn heart failures, should be considered to avoid energy/protein deficits.

Children's daily fluid requirements vary greatly, particularly in chronically or critically ill children. Depending on their elimination pattern, sweating, vomiting, fever, salivation, and age, daily fluid requirement varies from 130 to 40 ml/kg/day. Before even thinking of reducing fluids, we use the prescription of the attending physician. Nephrologists as well as cardiologists know very well how much is essentially needed. The threat of dehydration in MFCs is always present. In the chapters on tube weaning, we elaborate about this "danger." As a precursor, we remember using tests like specific weight of urine for assessment of dehydration. We concluded throughout the years that the urine collection in infants is quite intrusive (attaching urine collector sacks in girls, using catheters to collect urine from the bladder, etc.). We changed our approach by just looking at the child: does its mouth have sufficient saliva, can it close its eyes, what color of urine is seen in the diaper or toilet? Knowing this, and eventually seeing the child lust for liquid, which its mother or sibling drinks, is sufficient in all cases without a strict prescription of fluid intake.

According to the consensus of the Europe Society for Pediatric Gastroenterology, Hepatology and Nutrition's (ESPGHAN) Committee on Nutrition 2010 [4], standardized formulas are preferable to self-made food. The main arguments are better calculability, reduced tube clogging, and potential outcome evaluation and comparability in large populations of children receiving ENS. Highly specific formulas are needed for metabolic disorders, as well as periodic clinical assessment and accompanied lab tests which are compulsory to ensure efficacy of ENS.

If the body's length cannot be measured easily in severely handicapped children, the arm span, tibia length, or biceps circumference provides valid data. The ability to tolerate ENS varies greatly, depending on age, eventually GERD, gut tolerance and motility, general mobility, and the underlying medical disease. Standardized calculations of nutritional volumes and caloric value must be adapted individually. In a general population, thin people tend to eat frequently small portions, whereas obese people can eat great portions at any time. They may be less sensitive than lean people to environmental factors such as atmosphere, taste, style of serving, and the social situation. These individual variables also count for tube feeding. Some infants will require continuous tube feeds during the day, while some might tolerate tube feeds during their sleep better. Some manage boluses up to 250-300mls at a time, while some can't cope with more than 30mls/session. This might be related to medical issues like reflux or muscle tone affecting posture, but basically, it's the individual sensitivity to content and volume and can't be foreseen and demands individual experimenting.

In the lively discussion on the issue of blended food versus tube formula, we would like to remind readers of the times before medical science. In the early days of enteral nutrition, enemas were made. Food injected into the rectum consisted of purée or liquids: barley broth, soups, wine, sheep's milk, buttermilk, melted fat, butter, olive oil, egg yolks, and cow's milk. Discoveries in physiology found that the stomach is the organ one must place food into. Blended food was administered via orally inserted silver stomach tubes and then through syringes. In the twentieth century, Witzel invented a surgically made fistula, which held the stomach open and allowed the feeding of terminally ill patients directly with a spoon. Historically tubes were made from different materials such as leather and rubber. With the invention of plastic tubes which made from silicon or polyurethane, different types of tubes were developed, which made it possible to feed patients who, for example, suffered from esophageal atresia. Justus von Liebig invented a nutrition made for the adequate artificial feeding of newborns in 1866. Liebig's original soup recipe consisted of cow's milk, wheat and malt flour, and potassium carbonate. Using this soup, it was possible for the infants to survive, whose mothers couldn't breastfeed and couldn't afford a wet nurse. Until then, babies died because they were fed with goat milk (anemia was the consequence) or by cow's milk alone, which led to massive resorption problems.

As the German proverb goes: "He, who has the choice, has the torment." ("Wer die Wahl hat, hat die Qual)!" This also applies to the variety of ENS. Ever since mankind reached orbit and landed on the moon in 1969, it became necessary to manufacture a specific diet for astronauts [5]. The first astronauts only had dry bisques, but this insufficient diet had to be standardized and optimized. Astronauts spend months in space dealing with their metabolisms without gravity. Food must be effective, with long storage potential, high-calorie density, and excellent gut resorption, resulting in limited amount of feces. Astronaut food became available to the medical system, and in the early 1980s, the first PEG tube was inserted, making feeding in a lot of diagnoses which required adequate nutrition [6] much easier. The new way of feeding made it possible to optimize nutrition, for example, in preterm babies. The calculation of nutrition became easier and more accurate. The risks of homemade blended food are insufficient calories per quantity, wrong composition of food (mostly too little protein), lack of vitamins due to long cooking time, and too little variety of nutrients eventually lacking essential amino acids or fatty acids.

Possible arguments and advantages of blended food are that it's cheaper than tube formula and it gives more satisfaction to parents because they feel that they are feeding their child themselves as if it would be on a normal child. The urge to want to prepare food for one's child is instinctual. Blended food gives an impression of normality. Some children tolerate blended food better than tube formula, but dieticians propose the standardized formulas because of safety and because of what they are taught.

Disadvantages of blended food are that the preparation relies on good hygiene and ingredients should be of high quality. Because it has more fibrous texture than the industrially made nutrition, blended food might cause blockages of the feeding tube. Additionally, the perishable nature of food ingredients (especially proteins like egg yolk and fish) must be observed.

Arguments in favor of standardized tube formula surround how it varies in calories contained in each volume. Formulas are divers in respect to energy density, ranging from 0.67 to 2 kcal/ml. Ingredients are proteins, fats, minerals, vitamins, fibers, minerals, and water—everything a child needs. The dietician as part of the team recommends what should be used. Not every tube feeding formula works well for every child. Some children tolerate the initially recommended tube feeding formula well, while in others, several tube feeding formulas must be tried until the nutrition does not cause side effects, such as retching or even vomiting. A cautious approach to tube feeding formulas tailored to each child is advisable, since in some cases, side effects such as diarrhea, strong reflux, gagging, and regurgitation can occur and tend to make weight gain and subsequently thriving impossible.

Pro arguments for industrially made tube formulas:

1. Variety in taste, viscosity, density, nutritional and caloric composition.
2. Ability to calculate precisely.
3. Enriched formulas available, containing up to 2–3 more than breast milk.
4. Long storage possible.

Arguments against:

5. Sometimes not well tolerated.
6. High costs—not every health insurance covers the costs.
7. Some tube formulas have a bad taste, especially the formulas where protein chains have been broken up to make absorption easier.

Every child reacts differently to the composition, portion sizing, and timing of administered formulas. Tolerance and nutritional efficacy are caused not only by the nutritional and caloric composition but also by serving schedules, individual enzyme and hormonal metabolism, and gut variations in motility, passage, and digestion. Every recommendation and adaption should therefore be based on the individual reactions of the child. The nutritional status and possible side effects of ENS should be continuously re-evaluated during at least monthly meetings.

References

1. Quigley M, Embleton ND, McGuire W. Formula versus donor breast milk for feeding preterm or low birth weight infants. Cochrane Database Syst Rev. 2018;6(6):CD002971. https://doi.org/10.1002/14651858.CD002971.pub4. Update in: Cochrane Database Syst Rev. 2019 Jul 19;7:CD002971. PMID: 29926476; PMCID: PMC6513381
2. WHO Multicentre Growth Reference Study Group. WHO child growth standards based on length/height, weight and age. Acta Paediatr Suppl. 2006;450:76–85. https://doi.org/10.1111/j.1651-2227.2006.tb02378.x. PMID: 16817681

3. Hermoso M, Tabacchi G, Iglesia-Altaba I, Bel-Serrat S, Moreno-Aznar LA, García-Santos Y, del Rosario García-Luzardo M, Santana-Salguero B, Peña-Quintana L, Serra-Majem L, Moran VH, Dykes F, Decsi T, Benetou V, Plada M, Trichopoulou A, Raats MM, Doets EL, Berti C, Cetin I, Koletzko B. The nutritional requirements of infants. Towards EU alignment of reference values: the EURRECA network. Matern Child Nutr. 2010;6(Suppl. 2):55–83.
4. Fewtrell M, Bronsky J, Campoy C, Domellöf M, Embleton N, Fidler Mis N, Hojsak I, Hulst JM, Indrio F, Lapillonne A, Molgaard C. Complementary feeding: a position paper by the European Society for Paediatric Gastroenterology, Hepatology, and Nutrition (ESPGHAN) Committee on Nutrition. January 2017 – Volume 64 – Issue 1
5. See also https://airandspace.si.edu/exhibitions/apollo-to-the-moon/online/astronaut-life/food-in-space.cfm. Seen on 12/27/2018.
6. Harkness L. The history of enteral nutrition therapy: from raw eggs and nasal tubes to purified amino acids and early postoperative jejunal delivery. J Am Diet Assoc. 2002;102(3):399–404.

Unintended Side Effects of ENT

The explicit goal of ENS is sufficient nutritional provision (when a natural oral intake is not possible or insufficient). It can usually be met by using an adapted milk for the needs of a newborn. For children with intolerances to milk, suffering from metabolic disorders, or having other special medical conditions, the range and diversity of alternatives including fully hydrolyzed formulas is rapidly growing. Advice from dieticians is a source of helpful information. Therefore, it won't go into the labyrinth of nutritional optimization and formulas for specific requirements, as this is their expertise.

We will stick to medical basics: a gentle and gradual weight gain starting with 100–200 g/week in infancy, and later per month, is the goal. The pace of which expected weight gain is achieved and monitored is different in every country. In France it's stricter than in the Czech Republic, and in Germany growth charts are followed very accurately. Austrian doctors tend to follow the family's needs and are generally accommodating. The main difference between European doctors and doctors from the USA seems to be similar to crime stories. In Europe the main question when writing, filming, or consuming a crime story is the "motive" and why someone became a murderer. In American television series like NYPD, the remnants are analyzed on the spot, the evidence is collected, and the question of "why?" does not have a great value. It is the way it is. Man is man's enemy (lupus est homo homi-nem, T.M. Plautus 254–184 BC). The comparison may seem unrelated, but we can use this to understand infant feeding: Europeans deal with the interaction, lack of parental intervention, or the child's inability to react to cues sent from their caregivers. Americans analyze the inability to sustain oneself by collecting a symptom list and finding solutions to promote eating.

Sometimes pediatricians don't ask parents about how the child is feeling and dealing with treatments and focus more on charts than the child. We call that a technical approach. A holistic approach where the effects of ENS, adverse effects, and growth are seen in one picture is ideal. Sometimes a holistic approach appears to be more in the domain of alternative, non-scientifically based medicine than classic

M. Dunitz-Scheer, P. J. Scheer, *Child-led Tube-management and Tube-weaning*, https://doi.org/10.1007/978-3-031-09090-5_10

pediatrics. Since most pediatricians don't work from a social security basis in Austria anymore, it seems to be improving, because the MD has more than 3 min of time per patient.

The adaptation of tube feeding formula depends on age and the course the child takes on the percentile chart according to its birthweight. Depending on the duration of expected ENS, the underlying medical condition, the child's tolerance to quantity and content, and the developmental phase the child is in, a decision is made whether to proceed with bolus feeds or continuous feeding using a pump. Sometimes parents don't trust in the function of the pump or encountered that the connections of the cables broke loose and continue to supervise the feeding by getting up during the night. ENS is usually introduced in the hospital and demands daily monitoring. A few days after introduction, adaptation should be achieved, allowing the child to be discharged, but the parents must be instructed carefully on how to continue with ENT. In the beginning, we recommend weekly monitoring to make sure that volumes are tolerated. The family's daily routine also needs to adapt to the feeding schedule, especially when older siblings are present; the newborn baby on ENT changes the focus of attention enormously.

The best achievable balance between volume, calories, and timing needs to be decided individually, and, in this phase, close communication between caregivers and the feeding team is imperative. Although there are numerous advantages of temporary tube feeding, there are also disadvantages.

10.1   Advantages of Enteral Feeding

The most important advantage of temporary tube feeding is its life-sustaining nutritional support. A sufficient enteral nutritional supply ensures the thriving and growth of the child and its general development in cases when oral intake is insufficient or impossible. Children benefit from ENT because it allows them to grow, but a medical indication and definition of clear goals is essential before each and every tube placement.

10.2   Disadvantages of Enteral Feeding

Unfortunately, depending on the feeding tube used, in some cases, the intended effects on the child's growth don't meet expectations. The reasons for this are mainly volume loss by vomiting, reflux, or limited volume tolerance, which is displayed as retching and crying. The result is insufficient weight gain and often reduced or no oral intake. These symptoms make ENT a challenge, and tube dependency may develop. In the long run, this is one of the main disadvantages. Tube dependency is defined by child's inability or active refusal to start any food-centered activity like touching or holding food, licking, biting, and eventually tasting and even swallowing food after the indicated time for ENT has passed. Tube dependency can only be diagnosed if no medical reasons hinder the child to eat. This condition leads to caregivers developing codependence. They become dependent on tube feeds, and family life is arranged around the tube feeding routine. Within weeks, most children forgot how or don't learn to eat at all. A vicious circle evolves, which can lead to parents and children getting stuck in a seemingly endless and frustrating tube feeding reliance. Negative side effects during ENT are retching, gagging, tube dislocations, tube leaking of gastric fluid onto the skin causing skin irritations, granulation tissue at the entrance hole, and inhibited development of language, smell, and taste.

In one of our papers [1] on the adverse effects of ENT, we analyzed 425 enteral-fed children admitted for the sake of tube weaning between 2009 and 2013. Results show that each child suffered from at least two troublesome and unintended side effects including vomiting, retching, and gagging during and after being fed. Additional side effects we observed were a diminished or at times complete lack of hunger, sweating while being fed, granulation tissue at the entrance of the PEG, gastroesophageal reflux (GERD), and problems swallowing when trying to eat orally. All participants of the study were treated by us either in the telemedical program or on-site. The study shows that neither NG nor PEG is better than one another regarding the unintended side effects of ENT. The assumption that an NG causes less side effects than a PEG, which leads frequently to the installation of a PEG after 3 months of NG, couldn't be supported by our study.

In another one of our studies [2], the nutritional and growth status of 287 MFC children receiving ENT was assessed. Nutritional and growth parameters of children aged 1–36 months over 5 years (2009–2013) who were born as MFC were analyzed. When compared with World Health Organization (WHO) weight and growth standards, our results showed that 25% of children were malnourished/underweight, whereas 18% were acutely malnourished, i.e., wasted, and 31% were found to be chronically malnourished, i.e., stunted. According to the WHO, "Stunting is a result of long-term nutritional deprivation and often results in delayed mental development, poor school performance and reduced intellectual capacity," whereas "wasting in children is a symptom of acute under-nutrition usually because of insufficient food intake or a high incidence of infections, especially diarrhea. Wasting impairs the functioning of the immune system and can lead to increased severity and susceptibility to diseases and increased risk of death." These definitions stem from the world survey of the WHO and are addressed mainly to poverty-stricken countries. It is quite striking that in Austria, in a very standardized NICU, malnourishment happened, while intake was strictly monitored.

The high prevalence of malnutrition in MFCs who are receiving adequate medical support is keeping them at a continuous risk of developing secondary diseases, which compromise their quality of life and may lead to detrimental outcomes. Most children on long-term ENT either do not receive or do not tolerate the prescribed and sufficient amounts of food (= energy). This may lead to the assumption that ENT is unable to provide enough nutrients required for growth and development. Perhaps the solution should be introducing oral eating as soon as possible or at least not only monitoring intake by prescribing but by making sure that the intended goals are met.

When achieving catch-up growth in MFCs, dietary composition and maintenance of the protein-carb ratio appear to be very important. Decreased enteral intake is often associated with deficiencies of specific nutrients like protein, vitamins, and minerals.

The hypothesis of sufficient ENT automatically leading to optimal weight gain unfortunately does not prove true for all children. Reduced efficiency of ENT is mainly caused by an imbalance of beneficial variables and negative side effects, which may result in growth delay. Literature on the long-term outcomes of enteral nutrition in medically fragile patients is scarce [3]. Data is collected using home visits, and a randomized study shows that the effect of home-based aftercare can't be assessed when using short time data collection. It may be the case that the effect of the costly home visits can only be found in long-term studies. The neuropsychological outcome of MFCs is still under surveillance, as the heroic achievements of modern medicine may leave a heavy burden on parents and children, because life is strenuous and not easy to enjoy. Optimization of nutritional support and the structural embedding of the care and aftercare of these patients is an important avenue for further improvement of long-term outcomes of MFCs.

The prognosis of most health conditions correlates strongly with over- or under-feeding, and prolonged malnutrition might worsen a child's development as well as the underlying medical condition. Some conditions result in failure to thrive according to age, even though enough carefully selected nutrients by tube are given. Long-term tube feeding might not be able to provide the increasing amount of nutrition needed, which compromises the efficacy of ENT. Standardized tube management based on biometric data together with parents' feedback and frequent meetings with the feeding team is necessary to ensure the developmental benefits of ENT.

10.3   Conclusion

In medically fragile children, ENS medicine aims to, but cannot, ensure adequate growth. The main reasons for this mismatch are limited tolerance to quantities or content (adding fat in order to reach 1.5 kcal/ml may result in long-lasting satiety and food refusal), nausea, vomiting, gagging, and retching.

Therefore, ENT for medically fragile children requires institutionally authorized, structurally embedded, highly specialized, and individually tailored tube management and aftercare programs. They should include a regular evaluation of growth parameters and caloric intake, making re-evaluation possible, and, if necessary, allow a change of the feeding regiment. Findings from our studies [4] also suggest that any child on enteral feeding should be monitored to recognize the point where adverse side effects might outsize the intended nutritional benefits [5].

It can be stressful for the medical and nutritional team and parents when the expected positive result of ENT, specifically weight gain, does not occur. Doctors who find themselves in these situations start seeking probable and less probable differential diagnoses. Thus, the child may experience an extensive number of clinical explorations. There is a risk of parents blaming negative outcomes on the feeding team or turning against each other, because they feel lost and simply do not know what to do. The modern healthcare system does not have any other niche, where money and time are available in such generous amounts, as the field of intensive neonatal and pediatric care. Although well equipped, doctors, pediatricians, surgeons, nurses, and therapists are not prophets. Therefore, no one can give full security and definite answers regarding how the baby's future in the coming weeks and months. At discharge, the NICU predictions are about as accurate as the weather forecast for the next month. The best thing parents can do is to hold onto the reports and observations from every day of the baby's treatment, because during this time, a very well-trained team that takes immense satisfaction in working with the tiniest, youngest, most frail, and fragile patients will be accessible 24/7.

The life of caregivers has been turned, and they must learn about things they did not know existed a short while ago, and of course there is no way to prepare for one's greatest fears becoming a reality. Parents often note down diagnostic terms and look them up on the Internet, which can be a wild jungle of information, and find frightening search results. The term "complications" appears over and over, and they do not understand or accept that all of the possible complications seem to be happening to their baby!

Doctors strive to help and usually know what they are doing. Most of them made tremendous sacrifices and worked hard to become medical doctors, and they have surely learned enough from their extensive education, but sometimes people answer questions even without a clue about what is correct. When the older doctors went through their studies, tubes had just been invented. For the first 20 years, research focused mainly on aspects like surgical complications and nutritional outcomes of enteral feeding in rare medical conditions [6]. Doctors are trained to recognize an indication for a tube and can advise on the pros and cons of which tube to use, as well as calculate how much formula is needed—but when it comes down to side effects like nausea, gagging, and complications like excessive vomiting leading to food refusal, their expertise often comes to an end. Parents may understandably become more and more desperate as the weeks of enteral feeding increase and the child has not gain weight as expected. Parents will logically seek additional advice. A pediatrician, even if experienced, has usually seen only a handful of patients receiving ENS. Each doctor as well as each set of parents deal with the possibility of the child having a limited tolerance for ENT differently, and their experience with tube feeding-related issues is close to none.

In the cases of limited tolerance, the pressure of parental expectation increases, the infant's intake and weight decreases, and all parties involved become distressed and often turn on each other. A mother visiting a doctor alone with her tube-fed infant who doesn't thrive will most likely be advised to increase formula so that the baby gains weight, ending up with her feeling guilty and trying to increase calories by enriching the formula or adding volume. The dialogue between mother and doctor may become stressful and awkward. What is important for parents and all professionals dealing with parents or caregivers of children on ENS is to differentiate between fears concerning the child (which have their origin in the past and in recollections) and facts, which cause real concerns and the need to take action. Fears and fantasies are imperative and should not be overlooked though, because they have an impact on parents' daily behavior and the atmosphere around the baby. Unintentionally, fears seem to creep into the surrounding air and into the expression of one's face and the pitch of one's voice. This can prevent a tube-fed baby from receiving any positive or proud responses from its mother or father, particularly in moments of flourishing and attempting to fulfill the parents' expectations with all its power.

Even if the phase of ENS is witnessed as being stressful, the idea of stopping ENS often provokes additional anxieties. After a period of shock, parents adapt and get used to all the drips, tubes, and monitors, and nurses and doctors continuously try to explain everything. After a while one becomes accustomed to the environment, although at first it seems impossible and overwhelming. The parents' role in the first phase of intensive care is to trust, visit, care, and love, but not to be fully responsible. Once everyone is out of the hospital and arrives at home, everything changes. No more monitors, no more nurses and medical rounds, just lots of time on their own. Then the issue of wanting and needing to feed the baby arises, which has been out of their hands up to this point and taken care of by competent medical staff using a tube and a feeding routine. When the medical team in charge for tube placement is not interested in any kind of further tube management issues, parents might feel especially defeated about their baby learning to eat orally. One seems to adapt and get used to difficult or even dreadful situations, but changing them might seem even more daunting. When the baby is receiving the tube, professionals ease anxiety by talking about this being temporary, necessary, and good, but after, parents feel lost and alone when it comes to issues of management and how to proceed. Unfortunately, many professionals who are involved in tube placement do not have the comprehension of how to end the temporary intervention.

References

1. Pahsini K, Marinschek S, Khan Z, Dunitz-Scheer M, Scheer PJ. Unintended adverse effects of enteral nutrition support: parental perspective. J Pediatr Gastroenterol Nutr. 2016;62(1):169–73. https://doi.org/10.1097/MPG.0000000000000919. PMID: 26704669
2. Khan Z, Marinschek S, Pahsini K, Scheer P, Morris N, Urlesberger B, Dunitz-Scheer M. Nutritional/growth status in a large cohort of medically fragile children receiving long-term enteral nutrition support. J Pediatr Gastroenterol Nutr. 2016;62(1):157–60. https://doi.org/10.1097/MPG.0000000000000931. PMID: 26237372
3. Parker G, Bhakta P, Lovett C, Olsen R, Paisley S, Turner D. Paediatric home care: a systematic review of randomized trials on costs and effectiveness. J Health Serv Res Policy. 2006;11(2):110–9. https://doi.org/10.1258/135581906776318947. PMID: 16608587
4. Sadeh-Kon T, Fradkin A, Dunitz-Scheer M, Golik-Guz T, Sarig-Klein R, David M, Weiss B, Sinai T. Long term nutritional and growth outcomes of children completing an intensive multidisciplinary tube-feeding weaning program. Clin Nutr. 2020;39(10):3153–9. https://doi.org/10.1016/j.clnu.2020.02.006. Epub 2020 Feb 15. PMID: 32107059

5. Shalem T, Fradkin A, Dunitz-Scheer M, Sadeh-Kon T, Goz-Gulik T, Fishler Y, Weiss B. Gastrostomy tube weaning and treatment of severe selective eating in childhood: experience in Israel using an intensive three week program. Isr Med Assoc J. 2016;18(6):331–5. PMID: 27468525

6. Joffe A, Anton N, Lequier L, Vandermeer B, Tjosvold L, Larsen B, Hartling L. Nutritional support for critically ill children. Cochrane Database Syst Rev. 2016;2016(5):CD005144. https://doi.org/10.1002/14651858.CD005144.pub3. PMID: 27230550; PMCID: PMC6517095

How, when, what, who, how much, what effects, which side effects, etc. are what this chapter is going to elucidate. When meeting a child who has been on ENT for more than a few months, the child and its family have adapted to tube feeding. This adaptation might have become so good that ENS feels like a normal and matter-of-fact thing to do, but in some cases the adaption has not entered normality. This means that professionals will need to ask about all the details very carefully. They should be open to the description of diverse pictures ranging from relief to nightmare, depending on how the child has adapted to the situation. "The use of enteral feeding pumps is essential for continuous feeding and is preferable to bolus feeding"; this simple recommendation of the ESPGHAN CoN comment (2010) is sensible and sounds practical. Nevertheless, it might result in continuous feeding 24/7 and an inability for the family to leave their home. Therefore, any considerations about secondary effects of ENS directly and on a child's social life or on the sleep quality are noteworthy. Social disadvantages must be considered when looking at the "bigger picture."

When ENT is tolerated well and has an overall positive effect on the child's general well-being, growth, and mood, the only topic to discuss is the need for increase or a possible change of formula adjusting to the child's growth. This can be covered by a pediatrician, a nurse, or a dietician familiar with the topic. The meetings should be scheduled every 6 months minimum and should include a blood sample containing a simple blood count, CRP, electrolytes, a gas analysis, and additional tests if there is a medical need. When nutritional goals are met, parents and professionals should start addressing the issue of transition to oral feeding. This may start with oral stimulation, and a timeline for discontinuation of ENT should be planned.

Conversely, when things are not moving as initially expected, the situation is quite different. Malnutrition can lead to specific deficiencies of macro- or micronutrients and may influence growth and development negatively. Suggested examinations include biannual review of the child's nutrition and growth status, physical examination, regular venous full blood counts, determination of micronutrients,

© The Author(s), under exclusive license to Springer Nature Switzerland AG 2022
M. Dunitz-Scheer, P. J. Scheer, *Child-led Tube-management and Tube-weaning*,
https://doi.org/10.1007/978-3-031-09090-5_11

tube integrity, exclusion of GERD, and other medical or tube-related complications or symptoms. A recent study by Pahsini et al. [1] showed that ENT caused complications more frequently than expected. In around half of 425 infants on ENT, side effects such as gagging, retching, nausea, vomiting, and sweating episodes were observed. It was even more surprising that the side effect of vomiting was as frequent in children with an NG tube as in those supported by a PEG tube. The assumption that a PEG tube reduces the frequency of negative side effects seems to be wrong. The enteral feeding seems to cause negative side effects, which reduce the favorable outcome of the enteral nutrition support. In the long run, it causes food aversion due to nausea and retching because of an unfavorable feeling of "over-satiety" leading to vomiting. Children who vomit frequently get to know the taste of the formula given mixed with enteral fluids and react to these smells and tastes aversely even after the end of ENT while transitioning to ENS.

Another issue is the impact of ENS on body composition, which was shown in a recent clinical investigation, to be predominantly fat [2]. Since energy requirements of chronically ill children may deviate from healthy ones, the formula should be chosen according to the intended bodyweight and goal and not solely according to age. Additionally, fragile children show less movement than healthy ones. Energy will be converted mostly into fat resulting in even less movement.

Besides all the intended effects of placing a child on ENT and accepting certain tube-related side effects and complications, unfavorable developmental and social consequences must be acknowledged. Data concerning the psychological issues and emotional stress of tube-fed children is scarce [3]. Due to the direct relation between parents' emotional state and their behavior while performing daily ENT-related routines (attitude and mind set, preparation of tube feeds, rituals around the time the child is connected to the feeding pump, handling of gagging, nausea, and vomiting), professional attention paid specifically toward the parents' perception is of paramount importance. We observed all kinds of attitudes in parents. The tube seems to give parents a certain feeling of security. They know when to act and what to do. They feel safe regarding their parental chores, making thriving for their infant possible. Before, when still trying to feed their child orally, a lot of frustration and negative feedback from their doctors may have occurred. After tube placement and the prescription of the nutrition, they know what to do. When the child is unable to digest the prescribed amount, they tend to seek solutions such as extensions of feeding time or adding a food thickener. Only when a child does not gain weight at all irritation arises. But even then, doctors tend to assume non-compliance of parents.

When looking at the frequently reported symptom of vomits caused by gastro-esophageal reflux, the prescription of PPIs (proton pump inhibitors) to reduce the acidity of the stomach-liquid is not a causal therapy of reflux. It reduces the possible damage of the esophagus and heartburn and nothing more. Parents seem to believe that PPIs are a causal therapy of reflux, but they don't influence the motility of the esophagus. Additionally, they reduce digestion of proteins because they are less precipitated. Our own experience is restricted since we meet families mostly at the point when they have already made the decision to end ENT. We see exhausted parents, which sleep only for a few hours because they need to change a nutrition sack. We see children who don't know the feeling of hunger and satiety, and some even became averse to food when they smell it. We see families not able to leave their homes because they are sick of unsolicited stranger's comments on tube feeding. We see children whose social development and speech is delayed due to regurgitation and some other unpleasant feelings, neglected siblings where the tube-fed child plays the central role, and couples whose relationship is reduced to the duty of feeding without spouse-related functions.

The burden of tube-specific requirements can lead to restrictions of social interactions and personal activities of the whole family. The reported findings [4] on changes in parents' stress levels related to tube feeding and underlying medical condition are mixed. Some feel that ENS gives them a feeling of security; some feel that ENS is solely a burden and will try to replace formula by home-cooked tube feeds. A multidisciplinary team must detect parents who might develop ENS-related stress. We do not suggest that every child (and its family) on ENS should be referred for psychological and/or developmental assessment, but we feel that the impact of ENS on the child's general development should be considered.

Washing, bathing, and showering a child with permanent ENT is possible after wound healing, mostly 1–2 weeks after the PEG placement. To prevent material fatigue, a C-clamp can be placed and should then be repositioned daily or left open. The tube end needs to be cleaned daily with water and a soft brush, and the site of insertion must be kept clean, and the skin needs to be kept as dry as possible. Leaking of acid onto the skin should lead either to a change of the tube and without constant wetness of the skin because this may lead to local wound infection, which should be assessed and treated accordingly. Reddening of less than five millimeters around the skin stoma is frequent, but in the case of an infection, daily change of local dressing material and antiseptic measures might be necessary. In cases of a local infection, a physician must take a swab for microbiological examination and treat it accordingly.

Other local complications are tube occlusion [5] by the formula given (even more likely to occur with homemade food), which makes tube replacement necessary. This happens when the density or viscosity is inadequate due to the tube or the tube polymer becoming weak. The occurrence and severity of these complications are directly linked to the quality of aftercare and can be avoided if regular checkups are scheduled.

Regular meetings with the feeding team of the child receiving ENS are crucial. Awareness of nutritional and psychosocial aspects, evaluation of the intended benefits, and minimization of tube-related negative side effects are essential during follow-up.

It is necessary to highlight the impact of ENS from the perspective of the child, its parents, and healthcare providers. An infant perceives the presence of a tube, and it is undeniable that the urge for and pleasure of oral intake drops rapidly and often comes to a complete stop having lost hunger and thus any interest in nutrition. This is due to the constant externally regulated "fillings" producing saturation or even nausea and subsequently an absence of the sights, smells, and tastes of food. Once tube feeding has become established, every day may be spent balancing the aims of getting sufficient nutrition with the risk of side effects.

Some children will adapt to tube feeding and show sufficient weight gain, while others may fail to handle the volumes needed to obtain sufficient calories, and the time intervals between feeds feel too short for them, resulting in nausea or even vomiting. In some cases, tube feeding may alter the release of pancreatic enzymes [6] needed to absorb proteins and fats or change release of bowel hormones and reduce peristalsis. Affected children may fail to reach their weight or growth targets and may even show display food aversion.

The first feeling for parents after tube placement is often one of relief and diminished stress. Their child is finally receiving the valuable nutrients they need and, if food aversion is the reason for the tube, they can now have a break from the hours of feeding trials and seeing their child refusing every attempt at meal sessions, giving them the feeling that they are failing as parents. During the first days and weeks, constant support and availability by the medical team or a specifically assigned feeding team is advisable, to take care of all questions concerning the tube feeding, choice of formula, volumes, and technique and addressing side effects. The goal at that moment is to help the child continue to thrive, meeting its growth targets, and offering advice on how to maintain interest in oral feeding until the goals of a temporary intervention are met. The feeding team may then—after a period of weight gain—suggest an exit strategy from ENT, and the child can learn to eat orally. Some families may feel abandoned by the medical team with very little support and advice, particularly when a child doesn't benefit from the tube weight-wise and suffers from severe side effects. The best solution is to try to withhold the development of tube dependency, a situation where Notube has extensive experience and can be of help.

The requirements and quality of involvement during the phase of tube management can vary immensely for medical professionals. When the child tolerates tube feeding well and succeeds in meeting the intended targets with minimal intervention, the feeding team may feel like true heroes. The child is thriving, and the parents are grateful. In this case, the only role of the team would be to monitor the achievements and change feeding rates or formula depending on the success. Nevertheless, it may take a bit of trial and error before the best regime is found. This is easier when families are compliant, and the team works together to reach the best outcome. During both of these possible scenarios, the child should be supported by a team of therapists when necessary (speech, occupational, and physiotherapists) in order to help preserve oral functions with the aim of a smooth transition to orality later.

Real trouble occurs when tube feeding does not show the expected positive effect and the negative side effects (recurrent vomiting, nausea, gagging, retching) outweigh the nutritional benefits. At this point optimization may occur, compromising targets for the sake of reducing side effects. It is common that when a family is struggling to make progress, they look for other providers in search of a second opinion, desperate for a better solution to aid their child. Seeing a child not responding positively, despite the best efforts, challenges even medical professionals.

Members of feeding teams can end up waking up at night doubting and being insecure about basic professional skills, and this can damage the working relationship between them, the child, and the family. We encourage both health professionals and parents to remember that the decision to stop tube feeding all together may be the best solution when it is proving to be ineffective and nutritional goals are not being met.

11.1 Specific Issues of Gastrostomy Tubes

A G-tube is a tube, which is inserted through the skin of the abdomen into the stomach to deliver nutrition directly there. Using the PEG (percutaneous enteral gastrostomy), doctors, nutritionists, and parents control intake of fluids and nutrition. They are calculated according to the child's needs for its metabolic turnover, growth, and development. One possible differentiation can be drawn between temporary and permanent tubes. Permanent PEGs would be recommended in deteriorating medical conditions, in palliative therapy, and in some inborn errors of metabolism where bad-tasting liquids should be the only source of energy. Temporary PEGs should be inserted in children suffering from hematological diseases, like leukemia, and before, during, and after lifesaving operations like heart surgeries. The decision made by the medical team in conjunction with parents depends on the goals and purpose of the enteral feeding and the child's underlying medical condition.

Common medical conditions to insert a PEG are:

- Congenital abnormalities of the mouth, esophagus, stomach, intestines.
- Extreme prematurity (oxygen dependent, no possibility to eat for month).
- Severe brain injuries suffered around birth or after.
- Heart failures needing operations on the open heart.
- Global developmental delay without progress due to brain hemorrhage.
- Neuromuscular disorders of progressive nature.
- Metabolic disorders requiring a specific diet.
- Rarely: chronic failure to thrive.
- Untreatable gastroesophageal reflux.

In all these cases, some children improve, and the preference for a PEG might be reconsidered. For example, children after their first heart operation might be able to eat and gain weight so that a second operation becomes possible. We ourselves published data showing that the assumption of the magical 10 kg necessary for a big second operation was done without evidence. To gain weight by oral nutrition is of course more sustainable and allows more development than keeping a child on the PEG just because it might lose weight again.

In number 8, failure to thrive (FTT), we suspect that the decision to place a PEG might have been a result of desperation on the MD's and parent's side. Looking back gives one the impression that problems could have been handled better, but we know that is not true. Nevertheless, we strongly recommend one administers, if at all necessary, first a nasogastric (NG) tube before considering a PEG. We advocate this approach because for years we thought that the PEG showed less side effects than an NG tube, but when looking into the data of our patients, we found to our surprise that both types of feeding show nearly the same number of side effects like retching and vomiting. The only difference being that in NGs, it's the plaster mark on the cheek, and in PEGs, it's the inflammation of the abdominal skin.

The so-called untreatable reflux (number 9) might be an inability to handle a child, or problems caused by an overanxious child, or an unregulated child, for example, when its mother used cocaine during pregnancy. All these children should not be treated by changing the way food is installed. Maybe interactional problems, regulation disorders of early childhood, or some other complication causes inability to feed and/or to eat. Extensive diagnostic processes by a multidisciplinary team must be done before administering a PEG due to such an assumption. It may well be that the child and its parents become tube dependent although the indication for the insertion had been weak. One might assume that a PEG, which was weakly recommended, is easier to wean than another, which was needed urgently. Pitifully enough this is not the case. The reason might be that the inability to handle one's child stays the same when not improved by therapist during the enteral feeding time.

Regarding point 7, we add that we have treated children on a "stinky" diet, like only amino acids, and they learned to take that liquid orally. Children get used to the smell and the nature of the liquid and find it normal afterward.

Speaking of ingesting "stinky" food, we must think of our reaction to butter tea from Nepal or eating dogs or eating the brain of apes, which are presented alive at the table and killing these animals while eating seems to be a big treat to some people. If only mentioning this eating habit made you nauseas, then you know that one can't imagine the taste and smell preferences of another culture. It seems understandable and a good adaptation that children can get used to nutrition, which an adult would reject. There might be a "slot" in which adaptation takes place between the third and the ninth month. The first author of this book who is also part of our team is so optimistic she thinks that nearly all children can learn to eat. Only the children suffering from breathing difficulties and need oxygen support are not taken on by us as patients on-site anymore, because due to the number of people in our Eating-Schools, viral infections of the airways are frequent, and these children— normally kept as a single child at home—tend to react frequently and at times become so ill that they need treatment in an ICU.

11.2 Before Tube Placement (Pre-PEG Assessment)

Preferably, any child's feeding team should include those professionals who are involved in the indication for tube placement and will be responsible for tube feeding. Usually, the team contains a pediatrician, with a subspecialty in gastroenterology, or more rarely a pediatric surgeon who will place a G-tube and a professional (like a nutritionist) who takes care of maintenance and eventually the tube exit plan.

It is necessary to regularly check the efficiency of tube feeding (does it lead to weight gain or at least sufficient nutrition) and its side effects at the beginning in monthly intervals. Later, biannual meetings regarding medical, nutritional, and developmental concerns should be sufficient.

Before the intervention, it may be necessary to perform various diagnostic investigations (X-ray, ultrasound, etc.) depending on the illness, which made tube nutrition necessary. As with all operations, on the day of the gastrostomy, one is not allowed to drink or eat after midnight (overnight fast). Some children will need an intravenous infusion consisting of glucose and electrolytes. Usually, the gastrostomy is performed under full anesthesia or deep sedation by a gastroenterologist (in Germany and England) or by a child surgeon (in Austria). Who is responsible depends on the specific given local situation.

The gastroenterologist prescribes the enteral nutrition afterward, which will be followed up by a nutritionist. The G-tube is placed using an endoscopy. A "button [7]" (a device without tube hanging out of the abdomen—only tubes are connected to the hole, which is closed by the button [8]) can be used after having had a PEG; it works sufficiently and may be superior since the child doesn't bear any tubes hanging out from the womb. The button could be used as an intermediate device between full ENT and oral eating if insecurity on the parents or MD's side is present regarding whether the child will be able to sustain itself (like in swallowing problems or severe reflux). The button can be opened to insert food and closed in between usage.

11.3 Aftercare, Maintenance

After the PEG is in place (in some countries this will be done on an outpatient basis, while in others the child spends 1 or 2 days in hospital after full anesthesia), the child can return to its daily activities. To teach parents how to handle the PEG takes time. In hospital, parents must learn to take care of the tube by themselves, especially when delivering food. It's necessary to decide whether bolus feeding or continuous feeding using a pump is preferable. The arguments for bolus feeding are that parents can observe their child during feeding and decide which quantity it's capable of taking in, but the child may start to retch because its stomach is full. The argument for pump feeding is that the child can't cope with a bolus and needs to get food continuously (even as little as 20 ml/h) during the day and at night. Some children are preferably fed at night due to less vomiting. Especially in children suffering from esophageal atresia after operation using an intercept and lacking any esophageal motility, this might be a good choice. In the end the decision between continuous and bolus feeding is a psychosomatic one because it involves doctors, nutritionists, and parents' attitudes. The wish to feed one's child (bolus) or the idea that continuous feeding will have better results, the anxiety concerning a machine attached to a child (pump), and other influencing factors like non-scientifically proven ideas may play a role.

The efficiency of tube feeding should be checked using parent's reports:

– How successful was their or their child's adaptation?
– Are any side effects present requiring the doctor of the feeding team to see their patient?
– The tube feeding should be reconsidered, and it should be decided whether the PEG is a permanent or temporary device. If it's a temporary tube, the timespan for ENS should be planned by defining the nutritional goals.

The head of a tube maintenance team should be a pediatrician or the case-responsible MD. The team needs to include either therapists with special tube-related education, whether that is a speech therapist (SLP), occupational therapist, physiotherapist, a psychologist, or a nutritionist. Depending on the child's main issues, the team may ask additional specialists if sensory and/or developmental problems occur. An individual support plan for each child could be arranged with the help of parents.

Since children being fed by a G-tube are mostly able to eat/drink by mouth, they will be able to receive small amounts of fluids and/or taste some nutrients, thus receiving oral stimulation during the period of tube feeding. This may help later when the tube weaning process gets started. Offering liquids or food needs to be discussed before to withhold aspiration. Whether that can be done depends on the underlying diagnosis (like in Pierre-Robin syndrome with a malformation of the mouth). Keeping up oral activity and inducing the tube-fed child's interest for food and taste though being mainly tube fed can be recommended during the whole period of tube feeding.

References

1. Pahsini K, Marinschek S, Khan Z, Dunitz-Scheer M, Scheer PJ. Unintended adverse effects of enteral nutrition support: parental perspective. J Pediatr Gastroenterol Nutr. 2016;62(1):169–73.
2. Kaimbacher PS, Wallner-Liebmann SJ, Dunitz-Scheer M, Scheer PJ, Cvirns G, Schrabmair W, Schned WJ, Hamlin MJ, Tafeit E. Subcutaneous adipose tissue topography in long-term enterally fed children and healthy controls. Coll Antropol. 2015;39(3):601–9. PMID: 26898055
3. http://www.shieldhealthcare.com/community/grow/2015/07/07/caring-for-a-tube-fed-child-top-ten-emotional-issues/. Seen 12/31/2018.
4. Hazel R. The psychosocial impact on parents of tube feeding their child. Paediatr Nurs. 2006;18(4):19–22.
5. See also https://med.virginia.edu/ginutrition/wp-content/uploads/sites/199/2014/06/Parrish-March-14.pdf. Seen on 12/19/2018.
6. Graham C, Hoyle M. Pancreatic enzyme supplementation for patients receiving enteral feeds. Nutr Clin Pract. 2011;26(3):349–51.
7. Novotny NM, Vegeler RC, Breckler FD, Rescorla FJ.: Percutaneous endoscopic gastrostomy buttons in children: superior to tubes. J Pediatr Surg 2009;44(6):1193–96. https://doi.org/10.1016/j.jpedsurg.2009.02.024.
8. See as an example https://avanosmedicaldevices.com/digestive-health/enteral-feeding/mickey-feeding-tube-kits/. Seen on 6/4/21.

The following section summarizes specific ENS-related issues of pediatric conditions. In a large sample of exclusively enterally fed infants, Trabi et al. [1] defined, in 2010, ten different groups based on the frequency of the assigned main medical diagnosis having led to the administration of nutritional support via feeding tube. Marinschek et al. adapted this original list to newer findings of our work which were published in 2014, 2015, and 2019. This classification makes even more sense and is based on impairment assessments [2]. Since most affected infants suffer from more than one "primary diagnosis," the assignment and differentiation of any diagnosis in any given child is based on individual selection and common sense. The WHO offers different points of interest on which the focus should be laid. In our list we used, the *Diagnostic and Statistical Manual for Mental Disorders* in its fifth revision [3] claims that its diagnoses are based on an assembly of symptoms rather than on causes in opposition to the WHO-based ICD 10 (International Classification of Diseases and related health problems [4]) which also covers causally defined diagnostic entities especially in so-called somatic medicine, but also in psychiatric disorders.[1]

The ten groups in which we divide our clients for scientific reasons are:

1. Complicated prematurity and/or birth complications.
2. Congenital cardiac malformations.
3. Congenital metabolic diseases.
4. Malformation/diseases of the GIT (gastrointestinal tract).
5. Genetic syndromes/chromosomal abnormalities.

---

[1] It seems striking that the composition of criminal series in Europe do look for the motive of the perpetrator, whereas US-American series look for proof and evidence and don't care at all for the thrive of the murderer, which made him or her become a criminal. (See also A. Pfabigan: Mord zum Sonntag, Residenz, Salzburg, 2016. https://www.residenzverlag.com/buch/mord-zum-sonntag, seen on 6/5/21)

© The Author(s), under exclusive license to Springer Nature
Switzerland AG 2022
M. Dunitz-Scheer, P. J. Scheer, *Child-led Tube-management and Tube-weaning*,
https://doi.org/10.1007/978-3-031-09090-5_12

6. Psychiatric disease of the child or parent ending up in non-organic failure to thrive (FTT) and/or infantile anorexia (IF).
7. Neurological disorders.
8. Malformation/disease of respiratory tract.
9. Oncology and hemato-oncology.
10. Renal problems.

Since each of these groups differs significantly in the specific underlying medical issues, they deserve special considerations in respect to the ENS and which cautions are to be taken when a child is affected by a specific disorder or its remnants.

The following chapter will focus on the diversity of ENS-related issues associated with diverse underlying medical diagnoses and conditions. It should be considered that nearly every medically fragile child who receives ENS is affected by 2–3 or more specific, but separate, unrelated diagnostic entities. The following section offers a summary of main aspects and highlights the characteristics of each group as seen from the perspective of ENS and ENT.

12.1   Complicated Prematurity and/or Birth Complications

ENT is closely connected to prematurely born children and the necessity to ensure the best possible nutritional supply for them after birth. Practically every child born earlier than 29 weeks or weighing less than 1200–1500 g will receive nutritional support mostly by nasogastric tube during the first weeks of its life. Human breast milk is the first nutritional option, sometimes enriched. In most children the transition from exclusive enteral to oral feeding happens gradually and gently, when the staff of the NICU is trained accordingly and the child does not suffer from additional medical complications restricting growth. Extreme prematurity is per se a risk factor for developing tube dependence later as Pahsini et al. showed in 2018. Oral stimulation is recommended by non-nutritive stimulation starting (provided that NO lemon swabs are used, which are aversive to newborns) as soon as possible when the infant is in a medically stable state. The transition from tube to oral feeding is supported by non-nutritional followed by nutritional stimulation gradually increasing to oral feeding at gestational age (GA) of 28-30-34, depending mainly on the degree of involvement and diligence of the specialized nursing team. In an optimal case, it can be completed successfully with ad libitum oral feeding before the child reaches its calculated birth date.

Prematurity-related complications have a much greater influence on the risk of being able to transition to oral feeding at the given developmental slot than the degree of prematurity and birthweight. We recommend teaching very-low-birthweight (VLBW) and extremely preterm infants to eat during their inpatient stay.

We have seen many children born prematurely. More than half of all patients (53%) referred to us with tube dependence were born before 36 GA, one-third of them before 29 GA [5]. We treated over 300 extremely premature children between 2009 and 2017 and helped them to get rid of the feeding tube and transit to sustainable oral feeding. Most of them were referred from centers outside Austria. Fortunately, the issue of early oral stimulation during and after intensive care is taken care of in Austrian neonatal intensive care units (NICUs) very well. The goal is to discharge all premature-born infants without a feeding tube. The indication why the preemies in our study group received ENT was clear in most cases; they had been too frail, too small, too immature, and sometimes also too sick to eat by themselves. Their birthweight was 350–1500 g; they received auxiliary ventilation and were closely monitored and received only small amounts of breast milk by feeding tube. Months later, many of the neonatal problems were resolved, and children could be discharged. They can breathe, some can walk, and fortunately most of them continue to develop. Some of the VLBW children will show residual problems like a retina disorder (ROP), a frail lung due to BPD (bronchopulmonary dysplasia), a movement disorder following a cerebral hemorrhage, or even digestive problems, which developed after necrotizing enterocolitis. Movement disorders after prematurity affect the extremities. Such disabilities are referred to with the words CP (cerebral palsy), spastic paralysis, or undefined movement and walking disorder. When the infant's brain suffers severe damage, the effects may lead to developmental and intellectual disabilities. Practically all functions can be affected by brain injury: movement, breathing, and bowel movements. We won't list all the symptoms here, as each child is individually different and may have specific problems after an extremely premature birth or no issues at all. What is crucial for us is that when a child is born prematurely, its lips and mouth should be activated in a non-nutritive or later nutritive manner right from the start, assuring that safe and calm breathing works.

12.2   Intrauterine Growth Retardation (IUGR)

Intrauterine growth retardation means that the child's placenta didn't work sufficiently to allow adequate growth. This disorder affects approximately 4–8%; Romo et al. found 5.13% [6] affected. Once detected it requires a close monitoring of the pregnancy, as malnutrition of the fetus may lead to complications. The cause of the disorder is often unknown, but risk factors may be involved. There are many reasons why the placenta, which is made by the child, doesn't grow and/or functions adequately. The placenta might be too small, be deformed, or have structural abnormalities. Problems on the mother's side such as malnourishment, infections, high blood pressure, diabetes mellitus, or toxins (e.g., tobacco smoking or drugs like cocaine) can lead to a reduced supply of blood, oxygen, nutrients, and supplements for the child. On the child's side, genetic disorders and infections may lead to IUGR - the term SGA (small for gestational age) has sometimes been used synonymously although it should be reserved for smaller infants without a specific underlying medical but more often genetic reason for being small. It means a child is too small and/or too light for the calculated gestational week, but many seemingly too light or too little children are small due to their inheritance of the size of their parents or grandparents.

If malnourishment starts as late as in the third trimester, it is possible that children show catch-up growth [7]. Therefore, some children are overfed during the first months to reach the same body weight as the expected norm. ENT may be prescribed for that reason alone. We see children with this type of therapy sometimes overfed and overweight and even nauseous but not necessarily taller. Catch-up growth may be overestimated because MDs and parents hope that a higher weight enhances development of intellectual capabilities. This might be true in regions of famine but seems to be false for children in countries where NICUs exist. Mothers tend to blame themselves for IUGR, leading to maternal feelings of guilt. Questions like "do I have enough hormones?", "Am I too thin or too heavy or am I not eating the right diet?", and "Is my smoking to blame?" are asked. One or the other causes may apply, but IUGR children seemingly need a high-calorie diet to catch up. We assume that catch up should be possible with oral feeding. Only a few children need a feeding tube to increase the number of calories they take in. The discussion whether children show delayed development when they are slow in putting on weight after birth is controversial [8].

The belief that there is a connection between low weight and impaired brain development is another concern. Data shows that malnourished to-be mothers suffer a long-lasting effect. Improving intelligence by overfeeding may not occur at all. Most papers originate from areas of severe and chronic famine and should not be applied to developed countries [9]. Most causes for impaired growth cannot be questions of who is guilty; however, the evaluation and analysis of possible causes may be interesting for research reasons. Every mother wants to provide her child with optimal support for development during and after pregnancy. Whatever causes IUGR/SFD, the child should receive food orally, if possible, because natural oral food intake is always tolerated better than tube feeding. It shows less side effects and may even lead to better weight gain.

If the child suffering from IUGR receives a tube, it's important to know if catch-up growth is to be expected and when enteral feeding will be effective and worthwhile. This can be possible when the child was only affected in the last trimester of pregnancy. If this isn't the case, any attempt to make the child gain weight by adding more caloric enriched food by tube may be futile.

Many families find a growing aversion on the child's side influenced by increasing doctor's orders. In the end, the whole family may be concerned only with weight gain. When children are supplied with a feeding tube and prescribed large quantities of food to catch up, the acute pressure to get such an amount of food into one's child may elevate temporarily, but the issue of overfeeding is mostly just postponed and not ultimately solved.

In Summary The special task for this group of tube-dependent infants is to evaluate if the issue of premature birth or other birth-related complications is "past and over" and the child was just "forgotten" on ENT or might have lacked suitable oral rehabilitation measures at the given time *or* if there is a trauma (emotional or physical) still affecting the child, its parents, or both. In these cases, ENT management and the later transition to oral feeding will need to be accompanied by intensive and sensitive psychological support!

12.3 Congenital Malformations of the Heart

Infants suffering from congenital heart anomalies and cardiac failure requiring large, early, and repeated surgery are often started on ENT immediately after birth and usually tolerate tube feeding well with satisfying nutritional outcomes in most cases. ENT is offered either exclusively or as a supplement, while oral feeding is performed simultaneously. In one of our studies [10] we tried to fight the verdict that children suffering from heart diseases must weigh more than 10 kg before being operated a second time. Therefore, we investigated the success of prolonged tube feeding in pediatric patients with cardiac diseases. We found that this group showed the best nutritional results and had the best prognosis for early and easy transitioning to full nutrition orally. In children with a cardiac diagnosis, as a phenomenon of a genetic syndrome, the likelihood of developing tube dependency is higher. When cardiac patients undergo many surgeries during their first years and spend months in the NICU, a characteristic motor delay can be observed as the child has spent most of its life lying flat on its back. Reduced muscular tone of the trunk, floppy arm, and leg muscles are typical with an impressive delay in sitting ability. This causes delayed biting and chewing abilities. These specific problems should be addressed while on ENT by physiotherapy which helps the child to practice a functional hand-mouth coordination as soon as food is offered.

A frequent reason for these children to develop a failure to thrive is the increased energy requirement due to heightened cardiac consumption. A healthy child's weight may stabilize when it becomes active physically by starting to crawl and later walk, although they should learn to compensate for this energy need. Cardiac children are often given a temporary feeding tube to boost their caloric intake before having corrective surgery. Additionally, lung disease, chronic infections, and thyroid disease can all also be present with failure to thrive. A current study [11] suggests at least 80% of children with failure to thrive also suffer from behaviorally caused eating disorders.

While tube feeding can be essential for a child who is losing weight or not gaining, we cannot stress the importance of diagnosing and treating the underlying cause enough and, if tube feeding is needed, continuing to address the aim of the ENT throughout the tube feeding process with clear treatment targets and plans preempting the need for tube feeding.

Summary The special task in this group is to differentiate between facts and fears. Many children receiving ENT after cardiac surgery are functionally "repaired" but might need special attention in daily life in respect of their specific cardiac situation. Others have spent months on intensive care and having survived show great developmental delays, also affecting their motor and postural capacities. Physiotherapy and the psychological support of parents of children after cardiac surgery is crucial and will also affect the process of learning to eat.

12.4   Congenital Metabolic Disorders

This diagnostic group probably poses the greatest challenge regarding predictability of ENT as a permanent or a temporary intervention. Depending on the individual specific inborn error of metabolism, and its specific treatment, the child with a congenital metabolic disorder on ENT might only need regular electrolyte and blood tests or could be at high risk for metabolic derailment caused and triggered by their disease. The degree of brain damage and dysphagia, as well as the taste of specific diets, influences the decision whether individually tailored ENT for the metabolic disorder will be permanent or temporary. If it's "only" a temporary ENT, then every measure should be taken to support the child's nutrition via tube, which should be given as shortly as possible. Even nowadays, the prognosis of some of the metabolic diseases is not promising; it might well be that joyful oral eating can be achieved even in children with limited life expectancy. Partial or complete oral intake may well enhance the quality of life for the child as well as for the parents who undergo a lot of stress. Recurrent anxiety and inpatient stays in the hospital with their child create additional stress. If tube feeding is expected to be permanent, then parents must be informed about that, and expectations that tube weaning will be possible should be denied.

Summary   This is the most diverse diagnostic subgroup of all. Some types of error of metabolism can be corrected and stabilized by pharmaceutical supplementation and, if detected early enough, allow the child to develop into an individual only needing support in learning how to eat.

Depending on the nature of the specific metabolic pathology, others will be severely and chronically handicapped or even in a state of permanent impaired vigilance. The provision of PEG tubes for this last group should be considered early, as it will be life sustaining, and hopefully a relief for the child and their family. In cases of severe ENT-related side effects like constant vomiting, additional interventions like Nissen fundoplication or other supportive measures will need to be considered.

12.5   Malformations and Diseases of the Gastrointestinal Tract (GIT)

Concerning the possibility of learning oral eating, the distinction between primary and secondary tube dependency is important. Malformations, which require immediate post-partal surgical intervention (we include congenital diaphragmatic hernia here, but mainly esophageal and anal atresia), need the right moment (Kairos [12]— the right moment in ancient Greek mythology) after recovery to start with oral stimulation and subsequent eating. There is no point in waiting too long because it's necessary to use the corrected organ as well as it's urgent to try to eat to withhold tube dependency.

The placement of a primary NGT or PEG in children suffering from congenital malformations of the gut might not be possible due to the specific anatomical situation, and in some cases distinct individual solutions need to be found. In such cases, a nasogastric tube must be considered even for extended periods of time until anatomical issues have been resolved. One must bear in mind that, besides the problems of taping an NG tube to the cheek, the PEG seems only to be advantageous. In respect to negative side effects, NG and PEG tubes are alike. If ENT is planned as a temporary and transitory intervention, the period and duration of the tube placement should be kept as short as possible. One must keep in mind that a tube given to treat side effects of oral eating like retching or vomiting may be misleading. These symptoms might become worse when tube feeding because the filling of the stomach might even exceed the amount of food before, and the mindset of the child, "I am looking forward to food," might be worsened due to the non-intentional being filled up by tube.

For children who suffer from late gastric emptying or an exocrine pancreatic insufficiency, ENT might not be helpful at all. The ability to digest fat-protein complexes will be as bad as before with tube feedings and the more the amount of food increases. Thus, enzymatic activity is more challenged and doesn't work better if the method of feeding has been changed. We observed in our sample of tube-dependent children [13] that after oral feeding was achieved, it reduced unpleasant experiences of feeding. The duration of unintended, negative side effects of tube feeding, which we published [14], may even lead to refusal of food because of the negative feelings these children have toward food, which makes them vomit. We therefore advocate that ENT should *not* be given, or if only for a short period, in children with a healthy gut for the sake of overcoming food refusal or infantile anorexia. These children need therapy of a multidisciplinary team addressing the psychological conflicts and not only nutritional support. In children suffering from anatomical problems, such as malrotation or atresia's, we advocate the shortest possible postoperative period of intravenous nutrition support, followed by any means by oral feeding. If a period of ENT via tube is necessary, it should be given only when a clear plan of oral stimulation and the transition to oral feeding exists. To learn to eat might add to these children's life quality and reduce side effects and enhance development in many aspects, like social competence and speech development. We strongly advocate to avoid negative side effects by eventually reducing the quantity of food so far that they don't meet guidelines. The compliance of parents, whose children underwent enteral surgery followed by unpleasant conditions (like dumping syndrome) after every feed, might be reduced. The hypersensitive postoperative children should be encouraged to tackle their nutrition as much as possible themselves—driven by their motivation, skills, and will only. It may be that empowering the child to eat actively might be more effective than following nutrition tables. We do see children fed exclusively ENT for years gaining very little weight although the prescribed amount of nutrition should result in a much better weight

[15]. Asking parents for explanations of this phenomenon shows that they stop feeding when retching arises or after vomiting. Compliance to prescriptions might be shackled. Sometimes absorption might be insufficient due to many reasons (not being hungry, not eating by oneself, misbalances of the microbiome, or other influences). Sometimes frank and open communication seems to be impossible between parents and doctors, reducing compliance further. Many families tell us that the nutritional team scolded them for non-compliance, which made openness nearly impossible.

Individual "gut problems "do not resemble one another! It is a necessity to differentiate carefully between functional, nutritional, enzymatic, and hormonal variables. Motility related-problems or microbiome imbalances, as well as stress-induced influences, may play a role. Many illnesses and psychological states are intermingled with one another. Detailed documentation of side effects, beneficial situations, and periods of gain and loss as an addition to precise "food diaries" need to be collected. Any changes in treatment need to be planned in a way so that the pros and cons of each decision are transparent and the risk of overlapping or confounding disturbances is reduced.

12.6   Genetic Syndromes and Chromosomal Anomalies

This group includes children suffering from little abnormalities to those with the most severe and extreme anomalies and pathologies even reducing life expectancy. For example, muscular hypotonia leads often to primary feeding difficulties, which, after receiving the result of the genetic analysis, might lead to a hasty decision to place an ENT before evaluating oral skills and swallow functions. These skills must be observed repeatedly in real time, offering the child food in a non-stressed environment by its caretaker. If a stable physical condition can be established and when safe swallow is possible, children with congenital syndromes and chromosomal anomalies should be transitioned as soon as possible to oral feeding. This process needs medical supervision by feeding specialists and if available Castillo-Morales [16] therapists. If aspiration due to dysphagia isn't a problem, these children don't need permanent ENT.

Another good example could be the Costello syndrome (a RASopathy) [17]. It's a rare disease in childhood, diagnosed approximately in 1 of 300,000 children. Affected children show characteristic symptoms such as specific craniofacial and musculoskeletal features, curly and/or sparse hair, loose and soft skin, increased pigmentation, general hypotonia, macrocephaly and various cardiac malformations, short stature, as well as various degrees of intellectual impairment. Although most children are born with normal weight and height, children suffering from Costello syndrome often show severe feeding difficulties during their first weeks or even months of life. The reason is unknown. Parents struggle to feed these babies adequate amounts of food. Children may be also diagnosed with "failure to thrive" already after the first months of life, which is considered the most common and challenging clinical problem in Costello children. Trying to feed Costello children adequately, even during repair of cardiac failures or therapy of other malformations, might become stressful for the family, which suffers already due to the situation of a child with a syndrome. Feelings of insufficiency as a parent may lead to psychological stress and guilt. Most children with Costello syndrome receive ENT within their first months of life. Gastroesophageal reflux (GERD) may also be an additional complication; therefore, most of the patients undergo a Nissen fundoplication [18], which eliminates the possibility of vomiting. When the acute situation of malnutrition has been resolved, transition to oral feeding must become the focus of treatment. The children we have treated diagnosed with Costello syndrome may develop tube dependency with common side effects such as oral aversion and food refusal very quickly. Although their state is stable from a medical point of view, the children fail to learn to eat independently. Children with Costello syndrome can eat and experience hunger and satiety, but the feeding team must learn their distinct needs, including extreme stubbornness and the wish to dominate their environment. We treated nearly two dozen of children with Costello syndrome using our online system (Netcoaching). Six of them started their voyage toward orality by attending our 14-day outpatient program (Eating-School). Nearly all our participants were successful in transitioning from enteral to sustainable oral nutrition.

Other common diagnoses of children needing ENS are Down syndrome, Noonan syndrome, and Cornelia de Lange syndrome (CdLS). We frequently work with children who suffer from rare genetic disorders. MDs are seeing these patients mostly for the first time. If textbooks assume (mostly with only very limited evidence) that eating is impossible in some of these children, MDs believe and sometimes don't even try to wean such a child from its tube. Scientific literature [19–21] seems to support this conviction, knowing that individuals with these disorders frequently suffer from eating and swallowing difficulties as well as a weak smell system. We recognize these papers and know that these children are difficult to feed. We also know that children suffering from choanal dysfunctions or malformations do have an altered or even complete lack of a sense of smell. We were able to observe the children in treatment with us and disprove the predictions of the teams who treated them before. It was assumed and quite certain that eating would be an impossibility for the children entering our treatment facility, but this was not the case. In both Costello and Down syndrome children, their personality and will power were extremely strong, and the refusal of food was tremendously firm.

To overcome resistance, our treatment model includes play picnics (where the food is played with, but not necessarily eaten) and playful therapy sessions focusing on the oral region (stimulating it with special devices, etc.). Including the parents is also critical, offering them counseling as well. What is striking is that despite their difficulties leading to surgeries and paramedical treatments, nearly all the children in our facility achieved a result of having the ability to eat. The duration of treatment varied between children, and telemedical treatment was necessary for a longer duration for some patients; therefore the ongoing contact with the team in charge of where the patient lived was essential. In addition to our interventions, the most significant help must come from their caregivers, which have trust and believe in their child. It is not at all easy when local doctors are skeptical and consider the limitations of these children to be finite. We highly recommend informal parent to parent electronic interactions, for example, Facebook groups, which we offer due to the limited number of affected children. To insist that these children may eventually be able to sustain themselves helps the people around them a lot. It is different from a basic hope; it is a belief.

Summary This group may exhibit an overlap with group 12.3: inborn errors of metabolism. The conscious knowledge of a specific genetic disorder may be beneficial or destructive to patients. A genetically confirmed diagnosis may have been found by chance having no clinical relevance, or it might explain a lot of symptoms and help to find the best possible help for a child. It may be "misused" to explain unrelated feeding difficulties. ENT is often started early in life after a genetic disorder has been found, sometimes too early, and without giving the child a chance to learn how to intake orally at their own pace and way of developing.

12.7   Psychiatric Disease of the Child or Parent, Non-organic FTT, Infantile Anorexia

The decision to start ENT on children with failure to thrive without any underlying medical condition requires close medical supervision and may not necessarily lead to the expected positive outcome. Hypersensitivity regarding a lot of different foods and the inability to eat adequate amounts of food and/or sufficient volumes of liquid limit the possibility of reaching healthy body composition again. Tolerance toward food and volume may be very difficult and thus limit the amount of caloric intake. Enteral feeding in severe cases of infantile anorexia [22] can be beneficial in the initial phase of acute malnutrition but needs to be discontinued as soon as possible to avoid tube dependence. The term "infantile anorexia" was introduced by one of our most esteemed teachers, Irene Chatoor, a Washington, DC.-based child psychiatrist with an enormous interest in infantile attachment and its consequences on eating behavior. Irene introduced the diagnosis of infantile anorexia, describing it as a behavior of an infant, which resembles the symptoms of anorexia nervosa in juveniles. Infants, as well as adolescents, refuse to eat, get slimmer and slimmer, and integrate their food refusal into their personality. Parents are stressed trying to feed their child and experience no success in trying to do so. As the "cause" of this disease lies in the behavior of the child, and the interaction with its environment, the treatment of applying ENT can be only partial and may reduce healing further. ENT is an intrusive way of feeding and this may result in the child experiencing many side effects and a detrimental change in the parent-child interaction, making force feeding in a way obligatory. The psychodynamics of the disorder may be overseen or neglected, and if so, therapy is reduced to ENT without addressing the relational issues between the child and the others. We recommend offering ENT only during an acute weight loss and use the time window created by ENT to focus on the causes of the disorder and apply psychosomatic thought and therapy.

Attachment issues and avoidance in relation to caretakers caused by intrusive feeding trials appear frequent but tend to dissolve after tube weaning has been performed and normal eating routines have been established. A study [23] investigating psychiatric morbidity in mothers of infants with feeding and eating disorders found that up to 85% experienced depressive episodes due to chronic maternal exhaustion and fears of the child reaching starvation. After successful therapy and normalization of the feeding behavior, the rate of depression decreased to 15%. Based on these results, it seems probable that most psychiatric symptoms are of a reactive nature in feeding disorders, and any kind of "mother blaming" should be avoided.

12.7.1 ENT and Autism

Autism spectrum disorders (ASDs) are pervasive developmental disorders. ASDs are characterized by impaired social interaction based on the inability of cue recognition, communication abnormalities, maladjusted reactions, and a disturbance of primary attachment qualities and skills. The term "spectrum" refers to a range of diverse expressions of these deficits. In 2021, the diagnosis of autism is made much earlier than it used to be. Nevertheless, it's still dependent on the awareness and the sensitivity of caregivers and experts. Many of the tube-fed children we encounter show symptoms of ASD. When infants are born extremely premature with a life-threatening condition, it results in a reduced interaction mode, where atypical ASD may be assumed. Genetic defects of various kinds may also show symptoms associated with ASD. The diagnosis may be not specific but have a resemblance of the symptoms associated with ASD. "Real" ASD becomes evident in infancy to early childhood but needs to be seen in a typical environment to be recognized and diagnosed. A child within the specific setting of complete isolation in a sterile unit within a NICU, for example, due to severe immune deficiency, may behave pathologically without being diagnosable. This does not mean they suffer from ASD, and it is impossible to have a differential diagnosis before the environmental impact ends. When children are growing up in a NICU, developmental and/or psychological assessment cannot make valid predictions. Deviant behavior might be temporary and just be an adjustment to the environment. It may nevertheless become part of its psychological pathway due to issues already present at birth or the impact of the NICU on sensory and emotional development. We have seen children leaving the hospital after more than 1 year with a relatively healthy cognitive, emotional, and social development. Others having been isolated for the same amount of time experienced negative impacts on their psychological development.

One of the early symptoms of ASD is the inability to establish eye contact [24]. Deciphering social cues, feelings, and moods of others, and understanding nonverbal cues and emotional states, are the symptoms that follow. These symptoms lead to difficulties in social interaction, making attachment to others a challenge, also resulting in reduced communication and impaired language acquisition. Children exhibit these stereotypical and recurring behavior patterns in play situations.

A special form of ASDs is the high-functioning/savant autistic spectrum disorder, formerly Asperger's[2] disease [25]. These children show an inability to understand emotions. Outside the social deficits, they typically have a special interest or even talent. For example, they play chess exceptionally well, remember a lot of numbers, even a whole stack of cards,[3] and might know sophisticated geographical or biological data in detail. Hans Asperger played chess with "his" children in the evenings, and the "Heilpaedagogik" (special education teacher) was in the basement of the University Children's Hospital. Children won frequently due to their talents although H. Asperger was an experienced chess player. His book on autism [26] shed new light on a disturbance, which had been seen formerly as an educational deficit. Specifically, the tendency to seek repetitive behavioral routines, and to be almost incapable of accepting changes in one's environment, or even to accept new clothes, had been seen as a limitation of the parents' education and a lack of a child's submission to rules. Furthermore, as those affected are unable to understand emotions, they cannot identify their feelings. At young ages these children don't know what they want or what they need, let alone what is going on inside them psychologically; they fear change. Fear becomes a predominant feeling for ASD children. Those affected often scream for hours after minimal alterations occur, such as a toy being put in a new place. The cause of the disorder remains unclear. Genetics may present an answer, but the pendulum goes from "it's all genetic" to "it's caused by environmental triggers" to a more modern combination of genetics, epigenetics, and developmental psychology.

The history of ASD extends back to the beginning of psychoanalysis in the USA after it was expelled from Germany and Austria as a so-called Jewish science. Bruno Bettelheim [27], Rudolf Ekstein [28], and many other psychoanalysts studied the subject closely between 1938 and 1950. They blamed the misconduct of the parents as a cause for autism and used psychoanalytic theory to explain it. Bettelheim had a technique of regulating the setting of his patients by allowing the children of the orthogenic school in Chicago [29] to open the doors when they wanted to go out, but almost no one was authorized to come into their rooms unless the patient decided to open the door for the person. Bettelheim called this the inverse concentration camp, having lived through Dachau and Buchenwald himself, where he was dismissed due to the help of his American affidavits. Bettelheim hypothesized that autism was triggered by family stress and specifically a lack of connection between mother and child. The idea of genetic causes of low-functioning autism (formerly Kanner's disease) is 2022 dominant [30]. It is most probable that ASD is a cerebral-organic disorder requiring a wide-ranging treatment concept [31] including brain

---

[2] We cite Hans Asperger being aware of the recent discussion about his involvement in euthanasia during the Nazi-regime in Austria. We refer to recent research showing H. Asperger as a strict obeying Roman Catholic man opposing Nazi race ideology. See also Falk D. Non-complicit: Revisiting Hans Asperger's Career in Nazi-era Vienna. J Autism Dev Disord. 2020 Jul;50(7):2573–2584. doi: 10.1007/s10803-019-03981-7. PMID: 30887409.

[3] See also the outstanding movie coached by a leading child-psychiatrist: Rainman https://en.wikipedia.org/wiki/Rain_Man, seen on June 17, 2021

stimulation and medication as well as behavioral psychotherapy. Psychodynamic concepts are not mirrored in literature as they lack scientific evidence and are more case-related reports mostly coming from France [32].

A multidimensional and holistic approach is what we find to be most effective, which includes behavioral therapies as well as medication and guiding. We oppose too highly structured therapies, which could be seen from the outside as comparable to breaking in a horse for a dressage or an elephant for the circus.

Many children affected with ASD have problems with eating and specifically with not getting sufficient nutrients due to their reliance on things not changing and having as little diversity in their surroundings as possible, preferring situations which are constantly the same. This can eventually lead to ENT. These children are frightened when they are confronted with new foods or anything different, so tube weaning is quite a challenge. They are usually highly selective with food and eat a restricted diet. We helped them to learn how to eat in an individually tailored setting and helped their caregivers support them. We started by introducing new colors, tastes, and textures, gradually and gently using a foreseeable structured plan.

12.8   Failure to Thrive (FTT) and why Can it Lead to Tube Dependency?

Failure to thrive is defined as restricted physical growth (height and weight below the third or fifth percentile or a decrease in growth across two major growth percentiles) consequently leading to abnormal growth and development. The cause of non-organic failure to thrive is inadequate nutritional intake [33].

In literature we find two terms: FTT (failure to thrive) and NOFT (non-organic failure to thrive). Failure to thrive can be a result of several reasons, and frequently more than one cause contributes to a faulted growth pattern. If age-appropriate infant and young child feeding (IYCF) practices are not followed, which comprise of meeting the minimum dietary diversity and minimum food frequency [34], there will not be enough calories to support growth. A child suffering from severe allergies or medical conditions like cystic fibrosis or celiac disease can also not be expected to grow within average percentiles. Furthermore, any medical condition that requires an excess of calories may also lead to caloric imbalance and consequently to a failure to thrive.

NOFT indicates that non-organic causes can lead to inappropriate infant and young child feeding practices and end up with a failure to thrive, for example, pathological mother-child interactions during nurturing, or a sequela of a chocking event, which led to food refusal and the child not being able to overcome the anxiety of swallowing afterward. In many cases, a psychosomatic association between physical and interaction-related causes intermingles and results in FTT.

There are warning signs which can help recognize failure to thrive in infants. In most cases FTT is discovered when children's weight does not increase, which is checked during routine doctor's visits. The diagnosis of FTT is met when the child's weight drops two major percentiles on their weight/growth chart. Normally the weight is seriously affected, and this is categorized as acute malnutrition, whereas stunting, meaning low height for age, is a sequela of chronic malnutrition. Stunting is more frequently present in underdeveloped countries as there is an intergenerational cycle of malnutrition, and the majority of the population is suffering from chronic caloric deficits [35]. The impaired development of head circumference, indicating insufficient brain development, is the last to get affected. We haven't seen reduced head circumference in NOFT, only in the one or two children who were also suffering from rickets, a very rare condition in developed countries because vitamin D supplements are almost obligatory. (Children's weights are measured and compared with WHO growth standards based on anthropometric data collected from thousands of children worldwide like the USA, Norway, Ghana, India, Brazil, and Oman. There are other growth charts in use nationally [36].) Definitions using the growth charts define failure to thrive as having anthropometric measurements below two standard deviations or the child being below the third percentile. Stunting is defined when the length/height is below the third percentile, and the definition for wasting is weight or length below the third percentile. It is worth knowing that most of the mentioned studies excluded low birthweight children (less than 2500 grams when born at term) and may not be accurate for MFCs [37]. Large for date children tend to grow closer to average growth rates and may appear to have failure to thrive when they are following their expected trend. A pediatrician will compare several measurements and charts, as well as observe the child eat; they will also check developmental milestones and physical signs before deciding.

A simpler definition of failure to thrive is malnutrition due to insufficient caloric attainment. This may be due to insufficient intake or supply, lack of absorption, or excess bodily requirements. Lack of food may be due to parental neglect or inability to provide sufficient food due to poor knowledge, the depression of caregivers, or poverty. The causes of malnutrition range drastically in different parts of the world. The United Nations reported numbers in 2019, and their findings were that most of the world's undernourished population lives in Asia and Africa, with 144 million children under the age of 5 being stunted and 47 million affected by wasting. These children are affected by repeated episodes of infection and limited nutrient intake. Although the United Nations launched the Zero Hunger Challenge in 2012, one in every ten people in the world is still exposed to severe levels of food insecurity, i.e., do not have regular access to safe, nutritious, and sufficient food [38].

Some children with FTT have physical challenges that hinder eating, such as cleft palate, neuromuscular disease affecting chewing and swallowing, and genetic disorders like Pierre-Robin syndrome. In other children, the root of reduced food intake is food refusal due to behavioral or eating disorders. These are multifactorial in origin. It is important for medical professionals to identify this and attempt to treat it before considering tube feeding. There are also children who are eating enough food, but their gastrointestinal (GI) tract does not absorb the nutrients properly. Common causes are celiac disease and other food allergies, which can cause diarrhea following exposure to certain foods. Additional disorders leading to FTT include short bowel syndrome, when a child is born missing a portion of the intestine or GI tract (this commonly occurs after surgery but can be congenital); pyloric stenosis, when the sphincter at the stomach is excessively large and powerful causing the child to vomit often; and metabolic disorders where the child lacks enzymes needed to absorb or process certain nutrients. It is rare for these underlying medical conditions to present themselves exclusively as failure to thrive, as the children are often unwell with other symptoms, but they do need consideration.

12.9 ENT and Neurological Conditions

The use and necessity of ENT in this group is widely accepted. In most cases, states of malnutrition in severely disabled children can be avoided by permanent ENS, and their quality of life can improve tremendously. Premature born or children born with asphyxia and later severe cerebral palsy (CP) often experience eating difficulties, particularly those with spastic quadriplegic and dyskinetic CP. There are multiple factors within this group that may lead to difficulty eating:

- Neuro-motor dyscoordination.
- Lack of oral skills, dysphagia.
- Visual and cognitive impairment.
- Lack of sensory integration.
- Pharyngeal and/or esophageal dysfunction.
- Severe reflux with possible aspiration.

All these factors increase the risk of malnourishment and impaired growth. Growth restriction due to feeding difficulties is a negative prognostic factor in terms of the survival of children suffering from CP, because it may end up in malnourishment and cachexia [39]. It has been shown that early gastrostomy placement is linked to better growth [40]. In regions with easily accessible ENT, especially for children with a very negative in GMFCS (gross motor function classification system, which has five steps from nearly normal to almost unable to move [41]) level IV, enteral nutrition can be helpful when the aim of therapy is the lengthening of the expected lifespan [42]. In such cases palliative and ethical considerations should also be discussed between the parents and the therapeutic team. The results illustrate that a sufficient nutritional status and growth on the low side of the growth percentiles can be accepted in children with severely impaired motor function, especially when they need to be carried and lack own motor abilities. They might benefit from early PEG tube placement, particularly when considering the association between growth restriction and premature death.

Handicapped children with low muscular tone frequently also suffer from severe GERD (gastroesophageal reflux disease) [43] and need reflux assessment and therapy.

12.10   ENS and Malformations and Diseases of the Respiratory Tract

ENS is suitable in situations where breathing is unstable, independent of the cause of the lung dysfunction [44]. The recommendations [45] of the ESPEGHAN for children suffering from cystic fibrosis, a genetic disease which makes mucus more viscous, show that sufficient nutrition is necessary for the development of the lungs in infants.

In study groups [46] of ENT children past the neonatal phase, the diagnostic category of pulmonary diseases is rarely the exclusive reason for ENT, although stable respiration is a key prerequisite for appetite regulation. Children undergoing lung surgery will need ENT until stabilization but will generally develop an appetite and be able to transition to oral intake once satisfactory oxygenation is achieved. It is important to be aware of the outcome of keeping a child on ENT longer than necessary, which is tube dependency. Therefore, an attempt to reduce nutrition to induce sensations of hunger and satiety is necessary. Discharge from the hospital while still on ENT might be needed but is as disappointing as dismissing the patient on auxiliary ventilation. The exact differential diagnosis of possible laryngeal instability and sufficient lung function is essential. This is noted because we have seen children where the ENT was the reason for being transferred to us, but unstable oxygenation was the actual problem and not the tube dependency. We are aware that mistakes and even failures happen daily in all medical institutions and generally everywhere, so we want to refrain from blaming anyone, as we have been part of the system, having made a lot of mistakes ourselves. We only want to remind colleagues that a second uninfluenced observation of reasons for inability to learn to eat might be an essential step in treatment.

A frequent diagnosis in our sample is a diaphragmatic hernia (congenital diaphragmatic hernia, CDH). This is a congenital defect in which the formation of the diaphragm is improper during fetal development. The majority of CDHs occur on the left side of the body, allowing the stomach, intestine, and sometimes the spleen to migrate into the chest cavity, thus inhibiting lung development. The bigger the hole in the diaphragm is, the more abdominal organs will find their way there. This results in a compression of the unborn child's lungs. Recent research shows that CDH does not only affect the lungs' growth, but also its overall functioning [47]. Approximately every second newborn with CDH shows additional bodily malformations [48]. A congenital diaphragmatic hernia occurs between 1 in 3000 and 1 in 4000 births, and up until the introduction of ECMO, death rates were up to 80% [49]. This defect is mostly diagnosed in utero with an ultrasound during routine medical checkups throughout pregnancy and, if possible, operated in utero right away. Specific further examinations (fetal MRI, etc.) define the severity of the CDH. The early diagnosis and planning of the best possible delivery—even when already operated—at a specialized perinatal center has a great influence on the survival of CDH children. With state-of-the-art therapy, the survival rate has increased to 70–90% [50]. When the diagnosis is unknown at delivery, these babies show severe breathing difficulties after delivery and are diagnosed a few hours later. All newborn CDH infants need intensive medical care. The treatment involves ECMO [51], ENT, or a nutrition drip, monitoring, urinary catheterization, and much more support. It has been observed that a surgical correction of the CDH after a preoperative stabilization phase of several days has been proven to be most effective [52] if antenatal treatment is not effective.

When respiration is stable and the child is recovering from surgery, it remains still for weeks or even months in the NICU. If children are on artificial respiration, they need ENS to thrive. The first months of life are quite intense for CDH children and their families. Ideally, parents get the chance to see and touch their baby as soon as possible, although the infant may already be attached to several devices. It can be shocking and even devastating seeing a baby with one tube in the trachea and another in the stomach, as well as a catheter possibly located in the belly button, all while the newborn is monitored by several sensors attached to its skin. During the treatment phase, the child and parents or caregivers go through a massive amount of stress, accumulating mental trauma as well. The child endures unpleasant measures it doesn't want to be subjected to and can't understand. CDH children suffer numerous oral traumas (repeated intubation, artificial respiration, suctions, tube placement, examinations, etc.), which might lead to oral hypersensitivity and aversion. Limited visiting hours, necessary surgeries that are still subject to asking for consent of parents, and additional caring for siblings or family are all serious stress factors. After NICU, a phase of stabilization at a hospital ward is obligatory. Once they are discharged from the hospital, children may need respiratory support at home. The typical window of time when the development of sucking and swallowing is successfully met is missed due to creating a prolonged need for ENT. A heart and breath monitor is prescribed and may be frightening as false alarms are frequent. Eventually support measures can be reduced, which in most cases will ease the situation. Although the critical treatment phase may seem to be over, prolonged post-traumatic stress disorders (PTSD) in parents, combined with the lack of oral development in the child, may lead to a feeding disorder.

Our focus and goal with CDH children is to end tube dependency, which can be a tremendous challenge to overcome. Thomas Schaible [53], the leading expert in CDH in Germany, refers many children to us who have not been able to master the transition to oral intake. The reason is that after ventilation and many other obstacles are overcome, the child gets stuck on ENT, and the typical timeframe of learning to eat has passed. Sucking like a newborn and rolling one's tongue against the cleft to extract milk from mother's nipple never occurs. The possible transition from breastfeeding or bottle-feeding hasn't happened either. When we see these children, they outgrow the interest in bottle-feeding and sometimes even spoon feeding, but they are competent children who know when they are hungry and point to their PEG when their mother has forgotten to supply their nutrients [54]. Tube dependency is frequent in CDH children. To transition them to orality, a change in the mindset of the parents and children is a necessity, and their attitudes must change toward the situation they are in. Parents must be willing to let go of their control of the baby's intake and quantities, and children must overcome their aversion. Hypersensitivity and anxiety regarding new and unknown food must change as well. Motivation to have normal eating habits rises due to a wish to participate in daily routines like school and birthday parties with friends, and on the parents' side as well, there is a strong desire to be able to send their children to day schools and camps. The transition is a slow process to overcome obstacles mostly involving "bad" habits, which both the parents and children have developed.

There are children who can independently succeed going from ENT to autonomous orality step by step if a good environment is given, but there are children who are not able to achieve this transition without specific therapy. Parents' reports show that the way out of tube dependency in CDH children might be hard [55].

12.11 ENS in Oncology and Hematology

Children with oncological or hemato-oncological problems require immediate therapy in which excellent nutrition must be assured. Oral eating might be insufficient due to the excessive caloric need. If bone marrow transplantation is needed, then the medications administered will ruin an extensive amount of tissue, especially in the oral cavity. This reduces the ability of the children to eat, and in some cases eating can even be harmful to their well-being. Most children are on ENT while undergoing chemotherapy and need to resume regular habits after the chemotherapy has stopped. When "hyper-nutrition" is required for therapeutic success, ENT and intravenous nutrition takes place, and as a result, children feel consistently nauseas. Another issue is when children have a compromised immune system and must be kept in seclusion with germ-free food, resulting in nutrition which does not have taste and the ability to taste is destroyed.

12.11.1 An Example

The oncologist of my pediatric hospital called me in because Fodor, a patient (already past puberty), was suffering from an aggressive recurrent leukemia and didn't resume eating after having undergone a bone marrow transplant for the second time. As I entered his patient room, which was sterilized, I started a little chat. I asked him where he is from and how old he is and followed with a few simple questions. He was from Hungary, from the town of Gödöllö, which led to a nice conversation about Queen Elizabeth, the wife of Franz Josef I., king of Austria and Hungary from 1848 to 1916. Queen Elisabeth, who Austrians like to call Sissi, loved the castle of Gödöllö, which her husband donated to her after they were crowned the Hungarian king and queen in Budapest (1867), and she considered the castle to be the best of all her accommodations. It was her favorite place. We started a discussion about the authenticity of this castle, as it was used as a children's foster home, a hospital, and a center for the communist party for many years, eventually being restored for tourism after the end of communism. At the end of the conversation about Sissi, I wanted to know if there was anything he considered possible to eat. He said that a Carinthian specialty named "Kasnudeln," a noodle filled with cheese, would be his choice for his first meal after an extensive period of time on ENT. He wanted to compare all frozen and pre-cooked noodles of that type. I was informed that I was allowed to use a small cooking plate in the oncology department, so I went to the supermarket, bought and prepared the noodles with a lot of creamy brown butter for him. Additionally, he told me that a game of football he played with my colleague, the oncologist Prof. Dr. Christian Urban, was a good memory because he admires him. We invited Christian to join us for that first meal. Christian ate with us and played with Fodor afterward for 15 min. We learned that the patient's father never showed up because he was unable to deal with the severity of his son's situation and could not bear to witness the frail appearance of his son who was formerly a strong ice hockey player. For a few moments, Fodor enjoyed the two doctors as surrogate parents. He started to eat, and we proceeded by tasting all the noodles on the market and talking about how in the future he would even be able to eat what was on the hospital menu, which he detested until that point.

A combination of psychodynamic therapy, cooking, and positive thinking ended a long period of food resistance and his inability to eat.

Placing children on temporary ENT is a standard procedure. Options of how to transition from ENT to oral intake depend on various factors, like the intensity of intraoral violation and ulceration of the mucous membranes, the role of the parents and caregivers, the preparation of food within the oncology department, and many more. Careful oral hygiene and gentle non-nutritive stimulation while on chemotherapy or undergoing a bone marrow transplant can help ensure a smooth transition to oral eating. For us, the main issues are the presentation of food, the emotional state of the patients while eating, whether companionship is provided, and lastly the quality of the food that may also influence the possibility of getting back to oral eating.

12.12 Renal Problems

Chronic renal insufficiency may produce a loss of appetite and may require ENS. The preservation of oral functions by drinking and ingesting small amounts of food during any phase of ENS is crucial. A transition to oral nutrition is only possible after the stabilization of the child's renal functions or after a renal transplant. Children suffering from renal insufficiency are often fed by tube, and the feeding tube is placed to maintain the child's stable fluid intake. Furthermore, children suffering from renal insufficiency often need to take medication with an unpleasant taste. For example, Aldactone-Saltucin is a diuretic that prevents the patient from experiencing potassium loss but tastes awful.

Kidneys excrete nitrogen waste products (BUN, blood, urea, nitrogen) produced from protein metabolism. For people suffering from renal insufficiency, nitrogens are retained and are poisoning their bodies. They cause the skin to appear yellow and appetite loss, and the treatment requires reduction of protein intake. Children suffering from renal insufficiency don't enjoy eating; the food tastes bad, and they are nauseated and disgusted at the idea of eating due to the poisoning they experience.

In cases of renal complications, these are the factors which often lead to the placement of a feeding tube:

- Lack of appetite due to an unpleasant tasting diet and bitter medicine.
- Repulsion at the thought of eating due to the inability to excrete BUN.
- The need to drink large amounts of fluid.

These problems may influence appetite or may lead to complete aversion. In most cases, a nasogastric tube is used at first, and then for long-term tube maintenance, a PEG tube is inserted. On several occasions, the outcome is the children not knowing what food tastes like, and their taste is influenced by their own negative experiences, the unappealing nature of the food offered to them, and a lack of hunger because of sufficient tube feeds. For example, if food is offered by a speech therapist (SLT), the children may react defensively.

If tube weaning is possible and attempted using an online approach (Netcoaching), the following steps should be considered:

Involving a pediatric nephrologist, preferably at a location near where the child lives.

- Discussing medication—medication shouldn't be the only remaining reason to stay on ENT after eating resumes.
- Deciding on how much fluid is needed.
- Defining the maximum protein daily intake—if it can change to a higher amount, then the variety of food can increase, potentially improving the taste of food.
- Involving a dietician, who could perhaps change the appearance, smell, and taste of food.
- Taking both the caregiver and child's situation seriously and respecting their views on the situation, in addition to the strict observation of the kidney function.

All those points help in setting up a treatment plan, which may eventually support tube weaning. The treatment plan should be tailored to the needs of each child with renal insufficiency as an individual. With a more multifaceted treatment approach, the child has an opportunity to learn what hunger is step by step and subsequently learns to eat. It is important to note that a plan of reducing ENT may bring up fears from the child, parents, or doctors and therapists.

At Notube we recommend home-based telemedical coaching for this group especially after transplant. The suppression of immunity makes telemedical therapy much more favorable, preventing infections, whereas in the "Eating-School" there is a risk of them occurring. An infection can significantly worsen the child's prognosis, which is why in this case, Notube's Eating-School and the hospital should be avoided. At Notube we have treated children before and after their kidney transplant and did not face difficulties we could not overcome, thanks to the help of local doctors and other professionals in transitioning them to autonomous eating.

12.13   Children Needing and Receiving Tubes without any Specific "Underlying" Medical Condition

The content of this chapter is not as straightforward as the issues we presented in the last section. The topic might sound bizarre, referring to a physically healthy child without having any medical history, being placed on ENT, and at times using a PEG for no comprehensible reason. How can this be? Why does this happen? Are parents and doctors negligent or does the health system lack the adequate support it needs to deal with these cases? Maybe certain children need a tube in some mysterious and undefinable way.

We will try to explain this unusual situation from a retrograde perspective:

The current use of a medical diagnosis—especially with the help of standardized diagnostic classification systems, such as the DSM 3, 4, and 5 (since 2013) and the ICD 9, 10 (since 1994), and soon 11 (1.1.2022)—suggests a clear definition of all kinds of medical issues, differentiated and tailored to every patient by using specific criteria of every organ system, their defects, and possible influences on metabolism and general health. This allows international research to take place and provides a basis for standardized communication between health system participants and medical insurance companies.

In contrast to pediatric patients after months of intensive care and support, who's medical history usually fills a dozen pages, we are now talking about tubes applied to (from a medical perspective) basically healthy children, and this seemingly illogical contradiction needs to be looked at carefully.

There are professionals who may prefer this chapter to be classified as dealing with the issue of Enteral Nutrition Support in healthy children. Colleagues justify the placement of tubes by using legal or ethical reasons, and it being necessary due to "mental or emotional disturbance." This explains the unusual finding of feeding by ENS in early childhood in these cases. Another quite common habit is to decorate a child with a term like "feeding disorder" or "early eating behavior disorder," placing the origin and cause of the symptoms onto the child itself or parents, especially if the mother can't cope with the stressful eating situation leading to the referral. Irene Chatoor [56], a distinguished adult psychiatrist, became aware of the seemingly forgotten infants of mothers suffering from postpartum depression and identified some common patterns in these infants in the early 1980s. Her six classification categories were published in separate papers, consecutively integrated into DC 0-3R (1994, 2005) and removed again in DC 0–5 in 2019 [57]. The original six categories written by Irene Chatoor [58] followed a chronological order and are listed here:

1. Feeding disorder of state regulation: Difficulties of calm coordination as seen in mother of infants with regulatory issues starting mostly already in the newborn period and often leading to failure to thrive.
2. Feeding disorder of caregiver-infant reciprocity: Difficulties of behavioral adjustment and sensitive dialogue between the baby and its mother as seen

especially in primary caregivers suffering from postpartum depression or other psychiatric illnesses (start age: birth to a 3–4 months).

3. Infantile anorexia, a clash of autonomy needs of the infant with the needs for control of the mother leading to food refusal and potentially life-threatening malnutrition.

4. Sensory food aversion: children are very sensitive to taste, texture, smell, etc. of food and eat only a very limited diet. This problem is often seen in children with ASD or children and/or extreme prematurity.

5. Feeding disorder associated with concurrent medical condition: This condition refers to the children with an underlying medical disease causing the eating problem or tube dependency.

6. Feeding disorder associated with gastrointestinal diseases and/or a post-traumatic feeding disorder: This disorder refers to children who had major aversive events or repeated noxious traumas in the oropharynx—such as a reflux, a chocking event, severe vomiting with the feeling of anoxia, traumatic acute intubation, or something similar.

These six categories were accepted as valid and helpful classification subgroups of cating disorders for professionals for three decades (1980–2010) but were cancelled in the recent revision of DC 0–5 and replaced by only three new categories differentiated by the amount the child eats: under- or overeating disorder and atypical eating disorder. These categories have the advantage that they reach a high interrater reliability but give no information regarding the cause or the specific troubles the child has which we regret. The new categories shed light on how the Zero to Three Association's mindset has changed, going from a psychodynamic concept to the mainstream American Association for Child and Adolescent Psychiatry, which advocates diagnostic categories in clusters of observable symptoms without an underlying theory.

Aside from whether we believe in the psychoanalytic theories found in the "old" categories of Irene Chatoor or the new ones in DC 0–5, we can help children earlier and more effectively if the physically healthy but functionally maladjusted children are detected. These infants suffer from concerning issues and sometimes severe dysfunctions and are referred to gastroenterologists, where they receive a feeding tube, because they don't gain weight. Some suffer from failure to thrive, but others show no physical symptoms.

We are not judgmental about possible reasons for ENT, but aim to understand the dynamics between nutrition, the tube, the child, and the feeding caregiver, which ensures a successful plan for a speedy return to oral intake. We use a family-oriented approach. Whether we use the highly effective online (Netcoaching) tool to counsel the family via telemedicine or our on-site day clinic in Graz, the mindset is always the same; we don't treat the "cause" of the disturbance, but access oral eating by supporting the child and family and allow the child to feel its hunger-satiety cycle. Our program relies on the ability of a child without an underlying somatic illness to eat independently, and we strengthen the self-esteem of the child and its family.

References

1. Trabi T, Dunitz-Scheer M, Kratky E, Beckenbach H, Scheer PJ. Inpatient tube weaning in children with long-term feeding tube dependency: a retrospective analysis. Infant Ment Health J. 2010;31(6):664–81. https://doi.org/10.1002/imhj.20277. PMID: 28543064

2. The child with multiple impairments. Paediatr Child Health. 2000;5(7):397–412. https://doi.org/10.1093/pch/5.7.397.

3. https://www.psychiatry.org/psychiatrists/practice/dsm, seen on 6/5/21.

4. https://www.who.int/standards/classifications/classification-of-diseases. seen on 6/5/21

5. Pahsini K, Marinschek S, Khan Z, Urlesberger B, Scheer PJ, Dunitz-Scheer M. Tube dependency as a result of prematurity. J Neonatal Perinatal Med. 2018;11(3):311–6. https://doi.org/10.3233/NPM-1799. PMID: 30010147

6. Romo A, Carceller R, Tobajas J. Intrauterine growth retardation (IUGR): epidemiology and etiology. Pediatr Endocrinol Rev. 2009;6(Suppl 3):332–6. PMID: 19404231

7. Toftlund LH, Halken S, Agertoft L, Zachariassen G. Catch-up growth, rapid weight growth, and continuous growth from birth to 6 years of age in very-preterm-born children. Neonatology. 2018;114(4):285–93. https://doi.org/10.1159/000489675. Epub 2018 Jul 16. PMID: 30011395

8. Takeuchi A, Yorifuji T, Hattori M, Tamai K, Nakamura K, Nakamura M, Kageyama M, Kubo T, Ogino T, Kobayashi K, Doi H. Catch-up growth and behavioral development among preterm, small-for-gestational-age children: a nationwide Japanese population-based study. Brain and Development. 2019;41(5):397–405. https://doi.org/10.1016/j.braindev.2018.12.004. Epub 2019 Jan 2. PMID: 30611596

9. Bhutta ZA, Berkley JA, Bandsma RHJ, Kerac M, Trehan I, Briend A. Severe childhood malnutrition. Nat Rev Dis Primers. 2017;21(3):17067. https://doi.org/10.1038/nrdp.2017.67. PMID: 28933421; PMCID: PMC7004825

10. Trabi T, Dunitz-Scheer M, Scheer PJ. Weaning in children with congenital heart diseases from nutritional tube is easier than in other children. Cardiology. 2006;106(3):167. https://doi.org/10.1159/000092844. Epub 2006 Apr 24. PMID: 16636548

11. Cole SZ, Lanham JS. Failure to thrive: an update. Am Fam Physician. 2011;83(7):829–34. PMID: 21524049

12. https://en.wikipedia.org/wiki/Kairos, seen on 6/12/21.

13. Marinschek S, Pahsini K, Scheer PJ, Dunitz-Scheer M. Long-term outcomes of an interdisciplinary tube weaning program: a quantitative study. J Pediatr Gastroenterol Nutr. 2019;68(4):591–4. https://doi.org/10.1097/MPG.0000000000002264. PMID: 30633107

14. Pahsini K, Marinschek S, Khan Z, Dunitz-Scheer M, Scheer PJ. Unintended adverse effects of enteral nutrition support: parental perspective. J Pediatr Gastroenterol Nutr. 2016;62(1):169–73. https://doi.org/10.1097/MPG.0000000000000919. PMID: 26704669

15. Khan Z, Marinschek S, Pahsini K, Scheer P, Morris N, Urlesberger B, Dunitz-Scheer M. Nutritional/growth status in a large cohort of medically fragile children receiving long-term enteral nutrition support. J Pediatr Gastroenterol Nutr. 2016;62(1):157–60. https://doi.org/10.1097/MPG.0000000000000931. PMID: 26237372

16. Castillo-Morales R, Brondo J, Hoyer H, Limbrock GJ. Die Behandlung von kau-, Schluck- und Sprechstörungen bei behinderten Kindern mit der orofazialen Regulationstherapie nach Castillo-Morales: Aufgabe für Pädiater und Zahnarzt [treatment of chewing, swallowing and speech defects in handicapped children with Castillo-Morales orofacial regulator therapy: advice for pediatricians and dentists]. Zahnarztl Mitt. 1985;75(9):935–42. 947-51. PMID: 2931921

17. Gripp KW, Rauen KA. Costello Syndrome. In: Adam MP, Ardinger HH, Pagon RA, Wallace SE, LJH B, Mirzaa G, Amemiya A, editors. GeneReviews® [Internet]. Seattle, WA: University of Washington, Seattle; 2006. Aug 29 [updated 2019 Aug 29] 1993–2021. PMID: 20301680.

18. Frazzoni M, Piccoli M, Conigliaro R, Frazzoni L, Melotti G. Laparoscopic fundoplication for gastroesophageal reflux disease. World J Gastroenterol. 2014;20(39):14272–9. https://doi.org/10.3748/wjg.v20.i39.14272. PMID: 25339814; PMCID: PMC4202356

19. Shah N, Rodriguez M, Louis DS, Lindley K, Milla PJ. Feeding difficulties and foregut dysmotility in Noonan's syndrome. Arch Dis Child. 1999;81(1):28–31. https://doi.org/10.1136/adc.81.1.28. PMID: 10373129; PMCID: PMC1717976
20. Parma B, Cianci P, Decimi V, Mariani M, Provero MC, Funari C, Tajè S, Apuril E, Cereda A, Panceri R, Maitz S, Fossati C, Selicorni A. Complex nutritional deficiencies in a large cohort of Italian patients with Cornelia de Lange syndrome spectrum. Am J Med Genet A. 2020;182(9):2094–101. https://doi.org/10.1002/ajmg.a.61749. Epub 2020 Jul 9. PMID: 32648352
21. Ravel A, Mircher C, Rebillat AS, Cieuta-Walti C, Megarbane A. Feeding problems and gastrointestinal diseases in Down syndrome. Arch Pediatr. 2020;27(1):53–60. https://doi.org/10.1016/j.arcped.2019.11.008. Epub 2019 Nov 26. PMID: 31784293
22. Chatoor I, Ganiban J, Surles J, Doussard-Roosevelt J. Physiological regulation and infantile anorexia: a pilot study. J Am Acad Child Adolesc Psychiatry. 2004;43(8):1019–25. https://doi.org/10.1097/01.chi.0000126977.64579.4e. PMID: 15266197
23. Dunitz M, Scheer PJ, Trojovsky A, Kaschnitz W, Kvas E, Macari S. Changes in psychopathology of parents of NOFT (non-organic failure to thrive) infants during treatment. Eur Child Adolesc Psychiatry. 1996;5(2):93–100. https://doi.org/10.1007/BF01989501. PMID: 8814415
24. Sanchack KE, Thomas CA. Autism spectrum disorder: primary care principles. Am Fam Physician. 2016;94(12):972–9. PMID: 28075089
25. de Giambattista C, Ventura P, Trerotoli P, Margari M, Palumbi R, Margari L. Subtyping the autism spectrum disorder: comparison of children with high functioning autism and Asperger syndrome. J Autism Dev Disord. 2019;49(1):138–50. https://doi.org/10.1007/s10803-018-3689-4. PMID: 30043350; PMCID: PMC6331497
26. Heilpädagogik: Einführung in die Psychopathologie des Kindes Für Ärzte, Lehrer, Psychologen, Richter und Fürsorgerinnen (German Edition) 4. Aufl. 1965. Softcover reprint of the original 4th ed. 1965 Auflage.
27. Bettelheim B. The empty fortress: infantile autism and the birth of the self. New York: The Free Press; 1967.
28. Ekstein R. Children of time and space, of action and impulse: clinical studies on the psychoanalytic treatment of severely disturbed children. New York: Appleton-Century-Crofts; 1966.
29. Zimmerman DP. Psychotherapy in residential treatment: historical development and critical issues. Child Adolesc Psychiatr Clin N Am. 2004;13(2):347–61. https://doi.org/10.1016/S1056-4993(03)00122-6. PMID: 15062350
30. Harris J. Leo Kanner and autism: a 75-year perspective. Int Rev Psychiatry. 2018;30(1):3–17. https://doi.org/10.1080/09540261.2018.1455646. Epub 2018 Apr 18. PMID: 29667863
31. Famitafreshi H, Karimian M. Overview of the recent advances in pathophysiology and treatment for autism. CNS Neurol Disord Drug Targets. 2018;17(8):590–4. https://doi.org/10.2174/1871527317666180706141654. PMID: 29984672
32. Bishop DVM, Swendsen J. Psychoanalysis in the treatment of autism: why is France a cultural outlier? BJPsych Bull. 2021;45(2):89–93. https://doi.org/10.1192/bjb.2020.138. PMID: 33327979; PMCID: PMC8111966
33. Larson-Nath C, Biank VF. Clinical review of failure to thrive in pediatric patients. Pediatr Ann. 2016;45(2):e46-9. https://doi.org/10.3928/00904481-20160114-01. PMID: 26878182
34. UNICEF. Infant and young child feeding. https://data.unicef.org/topic/nutrition/infant-and-young-child-feeding/. Accessed on 1.8.2021.
35. WORLD BANK. Prevalence of stunting, height for age. (% of children under 5 years). https://data.worldbank.org/indicator/SH.STA.STNT.ZS?end=2020&start=2020&view=bar, Accessed on 01.08.2021.
36. WHO growth standards for children. https://www.who.int/tools/child-growth-standards/standards. Accessed on 01.08.2021.
37. Zhang L, Lin JG, Liang S, Sun J, Gao NN, Wu Q, Zhang HY, Liu HJ, Cheng XD, Cao Y, Li Y. Comparison of postnatal growth charts of singleton preterm and term infants using World Health Organization standards at 40-160 weeks postmenstrual age: a Chinese single-center

retrospective cohort study. Front Pediatr. 2021;9:595882. https://doi.org/10.3389/fped.2021.595882. PMID: 33791257; PMCID: PMC8005644

38. UN. Peace, dignity and equality on a healthy planet. Global Issues/ Food. https://www.un.org/en/global-issues/food. Seen on 3.8.2021.

39. MacLennan AH, Thompson SC, Gecz J. Cerebral palsy: causes, pathways, and the role of genetic variants. Am J Obstet Gynecol. 2015;213(6):779–88. https://doi.org/10.1016/j.ajog.2015.05.034. Epub 2015 May 21. PMID: 26003063

40. Rempel G. The importance of good nutrition in children with cerebral palsy. Phys Med Rehabil Clin N Am. 2015;26(1):39–56. https://doi.org/10.1016/j.pmr.2014.09.001. PMID: 25479778

41. https://canchild.ca/en/resources/42-gross-motor-function-classification-system-expanded-revised-gmfcs-e-r. Seen on 06/21/2021.

42. Oftedal S, Davies PS, Boyd RN, Stevenson RD, Ware RS, Keawutan P, Benfer KA, Bell KL. Longitudinal growth, diet, and physical activity in young children with cerebral palsy. Pediatrics. 2016;138(4):e20161321. https://doi.org/10.1542/peds.2016-1321. Epub 2016 Sep 7. PMID: 27604185

43. Asgarshirazi M, Farokhzadeh-Soltani M, Keihanidost Z, Shariat M. Evaluation of feeding disorders including gastro-esophageal reflux and oropharyngeal dysfunction in children with cerebral palsy. J Family Reprod Health. 2017;11(4):197–201. PMID: 30288166; PMCID: PMC6168757

44. Piersigilli F, Van Grambezen B, Hocq C, Danhaive O. Nutrients and microbiota in lung diseases of prematurity: the placenta-gut-lung triangle. Nutrients. 2020;12(2):469. https://doi.org/10.3390/nu12020469. PMID: 32069822; PMCID: PMC7071142

45. Turck D, Braegger CP, Colombo C, Declercq D, Morton A, Pancheva R, Robberecht E, Stern M, Strandvik B, Wolfe S, Schneider SM, Wilschanski M. ESPEN-ESPGHAN-ECFS guidelines on nutrition care for infants, children, and adults with cystic fibrosis. Clin Nutr. 2016;35(3):557–77. https://doi.org/10.1016/j.clnu.2016.03.004. Epub 2016 Mar 15. PMID: 27068495

46. Barr PA, Mally PV, Caprio MC. Standardized nutrition protocol for very low-birth-weight infants resulted in less use of parenteral nutrition and associated complications, better growth, and lower rates of necrotizing enterocolitis. JPEN J Parenter Enteral Nutr. 2019;43(4):540–9. https://doi.org/10.1002/jpen.1453. Epub 2018 Nov 9. PMID: 30414179

47. Ameis D, Khoshgoo N, Keijzer R. Abnormal lung development in congenital diaphragmatic hernia. Semin Pediatr Surg. 2017;26(3):123–8. https://doi.org/10.1053/j.sempedsurg.2017.04.011. Epub 2017 Apr 25. PMID: 28641748

48. Zaiss I, Kehl S, Link K, Neff W, Schaible T, Sütterlin M, Siemer J. Associated malformations in congenital diaphragmatic hernia. Am J Perinatol. 2011;28(3):211–8. https://doi.org/10.1055/s-0030-1268235. Epub 2010 Oct 26. PMID: 20979012

49. Irish MS, Holm BA, Glick PL. Congenital diaphragmatic hernia. A historical review. Clin Perinatol. 1996;23(4):625–53. PMID: 8982561

50. Dingeldein M. Congenital diaphragmatic hernia: Management & Outcomes. Adv Pediatr Infect Dis. 2018;65(1):241–7. https://doi.org/10.1016/j.yapd.2018.05.001. Epub 2018 Jun 12. PMID: 30053927

51. Glenn IC, Abdulhai S, Lally PA, Schlager A, Congenital Diaphragmatic Hernia Study Group. Early CDH repair on ECMO: improved survival but no decrease in ECMO duration (a CDH Study Group Investigation). J Pediatr Surg. 2019;54(10):2038–43. https://doi.org/10.1016/j.jpedsurg.2019.01.063. Epub 2019 Feb 27. PMID: 30898400

52. Costa KM, Saxena AK. Surgical chylothorax in neonates: management and outcomes. World J Pediatr. 2018;14(2):110–5. https://doi.org/10.1007/s12519-018-0134-x. Epub 2018 Mar 5. PMID: 29508361

53. Waag KL, Loff S, Zahn K, Ali M, Hien S, Kratz M, Neff W, Schaffelder R, Schaible T. Congenital diaphragmatic hernia: a modern day approach. Semin Pediatr Surg. 2008;17(4):244–54. https://doi.org/10.1053/j.sempedsurg.2008.07.009. PMID: 19019293

54. See also parent report in https://notube.com/author/aureliecharriere, seen on 06/26/2021.

55. https://notube.com/resources-for-parents-and-family/how-i-found-my-daughters-way-out-from-diaphragmatic-hernia-routine. Seen 06/26/2021

56. Ammaniti M, Lucarelli L, Cimino S, D'Olimpio F, Chatoor I. Maternal psychopathology and child risk factors in infantile anorexia. Int J Eat Disord. 2010;43(3):233–40. https://doi.org/10.1002/eat.20688. PMID: 19350650

57. https://www.zerotothree.org/resources/services/dc-0-3r, seen on 07/05/2021.

58. Kerzner B, Milano K, MacLean WC Jr, Berall G, Stuart S, Chatoor I. A practical approach to classifying and managing feeding difficulties. Pediatrics. 2015;135(2):344–53. https://doi.org/10.1542/peds.2014-1630. Epub 2015 Jan 5. PMID: 25560449

Tube Dependence

13

Tube dependence as a "terminus technicus" was defined and published by us and our research group in two papers in 2009 [1] and 2011 [2]. The term describes a state of being "stuck" on the tube without a medical reason. When this is the case, there is no motive for the child to change from ENT toward a sustainable oral intake. Even if the child suffers from troubling side effects like gagging, retching, nausea, or recurrent vomiting, the type of nutrition will not change, as it has become dependent on tube feeds. The child becomes an unintended "victim" of ENT, and the situation is often described as a nightmare by the parents and family.

Here is a short **case history** of one of our very first tube-dependent children:

B., born healthy, was admitted to the infectious department of the University Children's Hospital in Graz at the age of 6 months, suffering from severe diarrhea in June 1986. She was isolated (as it was custom then), and her parents could visit her only once a week. The diagnosis of an adenovirus gut infection was confirmed. The child received infusions substituting electrolytes and sugar, but unfortunately, she was reinfected additionally by a nosocomial norovirus during the second week of her inpatient stay. She lost 1 kg in 7 days and actively refused all bottle- and spoon-offered liquids and nutrition. The medical team placed a nasogastric tube and started ENT. In the third week, B. developed hospitalism [3], which means that she regressed behaviorally and was becoming more and more quiet and depressed. The nursing team was unaware of R. A. Spitz's discovery from the early 1930s and advised parents (because the child showed bonding behavior when she saw her parents and cried and did not want to let them go) not to visit the ward anymore. For the next 10 weeks, ENT was continued with the aim of weight gain. Unfortunately, the child didn't regain any weight and completely withdrew. No eye contact, no smile, no hunger signs, she was sad and inactive. Understandably, the parents were distraught and asked for psychological support. After 3 months the child was presented to us with her parents for taking care of the psychological needs. The staff from her ward claimed that it would be impossible to nourish her by natural intake and that she had developed failure to thrive (FTT). B. had not gained any weight at

© The Author(s), under exclusive license to Springer Nature Switzerland AG 2022
M. Dunitz-Scheer, P. J. Scheer, *Child-led Tube-management and Tube-weaning*,
https://doi.org/10.1007/978-3-031-09090-5_13

all in the 3 months prior, on exclusive and well-calculated ENT. The gastroenterologist in charge was extremely concerned about her condition, and more and more clinical assessment was performed with suspicion of malabsorption or even liver failure. When I (Marguerite) met the family with their 9-month-old girl, she identified the deep desperation instantly. The three members of the family clung to each other and shared verbally and behaviorally how hopeless they felt. At that time, I had never met a child with an NG tube outside the NICU and intuitively felt that this small family needed to be with each other more than anything else. I called the director of the pediatric department and asked him whether I could dismiss the child immediately, and he consented. The child returned home with an NG tube, and I promised to see the child daily. Improvising, and having just experienced normal infant feeding with my own healthy children, I offered some unspecified recommendations such as offering soup or cookies if B. was interested, and within 4 days, the child could sustain herself, and the tube was removed. I continued to see her twice weekly for the next month, she steadily gained weight, and the relieved parents and the team asked me what I had done to induce the miraculous change. The main intervention was to solve the attachment issue of the three close family members and to see her daily even on weekends and evaluate her intake and weight continuously. I spoke to the parents regularly, encouraged them, and put the responsibility more and more into their hands. Retrospectively, the diagnosis was a reactive emotional imbalance due to prolonged separation after the initial medical episode, food refusal, and consecutive tube dependence. The intuitive decision to discharge them was the effective therapeutic intervention because the child could reassume her preexisting feeding skills within just a few days in her own safe home environment.

There was another child, who we met just 1 month after the one mentioned one above. It was an only 10-week-old infant presenting symptoms of excessive screaming since birth and failure to thrive with a clinical suspicion of an infantile regulatory disorder. The child was referred to the general admissions unit in the university hospital at the age of 6 weeks on a nasogastric tube and by chance was examined by the leading gastroenterologist on duty there. She decided to admit the infant for further diagnostic examinations, onto the gastroenterological ward all of which were of an intrusive nature. The child continued to barely drink anything, was tube fed, vomited, and screamed a lot. All examinations showed no pathological result, but the assessment took 4 weeks of inpatient care, and the final plan of action that came from it was a suggestion to do a liver biopsy. A scientific paper was given to the parents on fructose intolerance to explain the indication for the liver biopsy—a very rare congenital enzyme deficiency—and in this paper, 10 of the 12 children died. After reading this, the mother expressed wanting to jump out of the window, as she could not face seeing her infant die. Immediately after this event, the mother was transferred to the psychosomatic ward with suspicion of suicidal ideation, and we met an utterly desperate mother with her now 10-week-old child weighing only half a kilogram above its birthweight. The infant was visibly underweight while being fully tube fed and drank only very small portions of milk and vomited most of the tube-fed formula. She screamed when put flat on her back, but when she was picked up for comfort, she was happy and relaxed immediately, and with this discovery we decided that her mother should be the only person who picks her up and holds her. Any further medical examinations were forbidden with a clear note on the child's chart as indication for night shifts and the weekend team. We told B's mother to use her baby's short spans of attention to feed her little daughter compassionately. The tube feeds were reduced gently, and the tube was removed after only 2 days, because the oral intake increased.

The reasons for this positive development were:

– The exclusive feeding by the child's mother.
– The different outlook—respecting the mother-child dyad and seeing her as competent.
– The belief and trust that the two will find their own solution if we withheld disturbance.
– Continuously encouraging the parents.
– Reducing tube feeds while monitoring the baby's increasing oral intake and weight.

The mother and child spent 2 more weeks in our psychosomatic ward and were able to be discharged after good progress was made in drinking volumes and weight. Both these clinically impressive case histories were in fact very "simple" cases when looking at them from a medical perspective. What we learnt was how crucial the environmental influence and factors were. In the first case, immediate discharge from the hospital was the solution, while in the second case, it was very discrete and supportive inpatient support without any medical interventions at all. What both cases showed clearly was the ineffective, unnecessary, and potentially harmful solution of a temporarily placed tube. Both cases grabbed our attention, which turned into a fascination, when it came to the relationship between the tube-fed child and its natural caretaking system and the possible detrimental influence the health system has when introducing ENT to the child and family with the best of intentions.

After this, we had established a growing reputation of being some kind of magicians for infants with complex tube issues, and more and more patients were referred first from all over Austria, but soon also from Switzerland and Germany, as the pediatric community was quite close and not too huge in numbers. Over the years, the psychosomatic unit gained a good image, and in 2006, a BBC film team came to visit us for 3 full weeks and made the film "The Girl Who Never Ate [4]," accompanying a 7-year-old girl after successful surgically repaired esophagus atresia with her family all the way from England to Graz and back home again!

Ever since then, our name and fame has become the source of literally about 6000 tube-dependent children whom we met over the years with the aim of tube weaning.

Summarizing this unintended new clinical focus—which was supported in every way by the hospital and its administration—we can now state that the best and most effective preventative measures against tube dependence are:

- Placing as few tubes as possible and as many as necessary.
- Making the distinction between temporary and permanent ENT as early as possible.
- Offer a clear tube management/weaning plan for every child after tube placement.
- Define the intended nutritional goals as early as possible.
- Have every primarily tube fed child off ENT before the age of 12 months unless there is a medical reason withholding the transition to oral intake.
- Take care of and stimulate oral skills during all phases of ENT.
- When weaning is the clear mutually defined next step, do it if you have the means.
- If it does not work within 2–3 weeks, refer the child to an experienced and expert team in tube weaning performing at least 1–3 tube weaning programs monthly.

More details and e-books on each of these items can be found on the Notube website, www.notube.com, where worried parents and interested professionals may also use the option of a free evaluation of what they might wish to ask specifically.

Fortunately, the impact of tube dependence on four very specific areas of early development of medically fragile children was studied as a doctoral thesis by Hannes Beckenbach [5] in 2010 for the very first time. The start of his research was our observation that infants make an impressive developmental "jump" after being able to sustain themselves orally. At first, we were very surprised. Pediatric literature assumes that development is dependent on continuous sufficient intake of calories. This may be true for regions of the world where famine inhibits child development. In our clients, the negative side effects of ENS in combination with the impossibility to taste or smell seemed to reduce the child's interest in exploring its environment also on a general level. Explorational behavior is necessary for development as is a secure base provided by parents. As the feeling of not being well dominates others, most tube-dependent children's developmental growth is extremely limited. Beckenbach evaluated our clinical impression in an extensive qualitative study on 51 children—from 6 months to 3 years of age—assessing different regions of development. In his PhD thesis on medical science, he showed that ENS impaired development of four tasks: social learning, communication, empowerment to explore the environment, and interactional abilities. In all four areas, children leaped forward after having learnt to eat. Nevertheless, it did not affect intelligence in any way if protein and sugar was supplied sufficiently. After successful weaning was performed, all affected aspects could be improved in the study group.

The general impression of ENS is that it has a beneficial influence as increased weight gain leads to better motor activity, boost of immune system, and increased general energy in children suffering from malnutrition before ENS, regardless of its origin. Food given to children after exposure to famine, infantile anorexia, or gastric pathology making digestion nearly impossible will help but might not solve all issues.

Tube-dependent patients referred for tube weaning are a quite special group in various ways: either they have reached their nutritional goals, or tube feeding does not help them anymore, or they suffer from negative side effects which outweigh the nutritional benefit. This can become a major developmental and social issue since for one excessive vomiting will affect the child's and its family's quality of life in a profound way. Developmental delay as a side effect of tube feeding has been evaluated specifically by our group. Some papers (especially GM Craig who invested a whole researcher's life into that subject [6, 7]) report an increase in family stress, sleep disruption, and impairment of overall quality of life due to social isolation. The complexity of variables due to genetics, perinatal history, underlying medical condition, as well as psychological variables and coping strategies is immense. Information on developmental areas during the months and years of ENS, the impact of the act of discontinuation of ENS itself, and its influence on various developmental areas like speech, sensory awareness, and motor skills seem to be tremendous. After concluding Beckenbach's doctoral thesis and reflecting on it, we thought that perhaps the intervention in itself—including a multidisciplinary team and an inpatient stay for 21 days—could have led to the developmental leap. Since then—working in our "Eating-School" in a day care clinic-based model since 2016—we could observe that the developmental "jump" is as big or even more impressive as it was within the inpatient setting of the pediatric hospital.

Evaluating results of the exclusive online program in Graz, Austria, Sabine Marinschek [8] and her team could show that the weaning results of the online program were as good if not even superior on some levels as an inpatient stay. The only difference in respect to observation is that clients leave after 14 days so that the impact of tube weaning on development can't be observed if it has been in the hospital. Telemedical aftercare supplies us with video observation possibilities as do parents' reports using the telemedical system on Notube. Using this data, we are positive that the impact on development, which we saw 10 years ago, is at least the same [9]. Additionally, we could show that the 14-day intensive day clinic program at the Notube Eating-School was equally or even more effective as the 21 inpatient clinic programs had been, and the environment prepared in the Eating-School for the process demands less effort and adaptation of the accompanying families and doesn't remind them as much of their time in the NICU or any other inpatient stays.

The observation of growth and developmental progress due to the tube weaning process itself has not been studied in larger populations yet. This is partially because ethical considerations prevent studying populations of tube-fed children seeking professional support into any kind of prospective, randomized study when peer-reviewed weaning reports (like ours) offer a success rate of at least 90%. Another reason why the long-term care of tube-fed infants and toddler is often insufficient [10] is that hospitals and any healthcare institutions are more skilled in tube placement than in the management of ENT and in tube weaning [11]. ENT management demands high and intensive staff involvement and special professional respect toward families, awareness toward children's needs, and provision of support a child and its family might need. A child on exclusive tube feeds might show a mild, moderate, or lengthy delay of eating and drinking development. The longer ENT lasts, the more powerful the delay. The gap between the non-emerging eating behavior and its general developmental level will increase. This phenomenon may stem from oral traumatization and present itself as total food refusal or even aversion in otherwise well-developed children. In the existing literature [12] on the topic of complications in temporary enteral nutrition, the term "tube-dependence [13]" is referred to as the child's unwillingness, inability, or active refusal to initiate oral activity such as touching, holding, licking, tasting, or biting food, in absence of medical reasons to continue enteral feeding. We are proud that we invented the "diagnosis" of an unintended side effect of ENT, which had become unnecessary from a medical and nutritional standpoint. Nowadays, it's a common term and highlights the necessity to intervene to avoid additional shortcomings in a child's development. The awareness of the phenomenon of delaying or missing the development of eating behavior didn't exist much before 2010.

Prospective criteria for the risk of developing tube dependence are:

- Extreme prematurity (VLBW child).
- Severe developmental delay.
- Severe bronchopulmonary dysplasia (BPD).
- Phenotypically detectable severe of genetic dysfunctions.
- Intranatal complications.
- Postnatal complications.
- Initially temporary ENT for more than 6 months.
- Insufficient weight gain although on ENT.
- Negative side effects like dumping syndrome, excessive vomiting, gagging, retching, nausea.
- Repeated microbiological contamination of the enteral tube.
- Repeated traumatic experiences during intensive care and tube changes.
- Lack of non-nutritive sucking stimulation during ENT.
- Refusal and/or avoidance toward feeding trials.
- Highly insecure parents who receive insufficient support during ENT.
- Lack of intuitive parenting behavior.
- Enduring or episodic psychiatric diagnosis of a parent.

Our most frequent finding during the assessment of tube-fed toddlers is a nonexistence of eating/drinking-related activities often combined with delayed speech development. Some features of the DSM [14] V [15] describe feeding disorder based on regulatory issues, patterns of infantile anorexia, attachment problems, and sensory as well as perception issues, which can co-exist with tube dependence and need to be tackled when observed [16].

The enterally fed child never seems to express hunger cues. Olfactory and visual offering of food may be mostly perceived by the infant as irritating, intrusive, or even negative. The main reason for food aversive behavior seems to be satiety, because of too much food or too short intervals between tube feeds, which may be placed 3–4 h apart during day and night.

The diagnostic assessment of the oral readiness for tube weaning while still on ENS should be performed after at least 8–10 h of fasting. Food should be offered in a suitable posture, allowing the child to use its arms and hands while having its back firmly supported. The pharyngeal region should be positioned upright unless the child is severely handicapped and requires a supine position. The focus on the quality of oral activity and the infant's/child's willingness to direct its attention and hand motor coordination toward food seem to be reliable predictive factors for its ability to learn to eat.

The capacity for sucking on a pacifier might also give some hints regarding the ability and potential for sucking. By dipping the pacifier in water or 10% glucose solution (in children less than 1 year of age, the solution shouldn't be prepared with honey because of the very rare possibility of a botulism contamination [17]). Using sugar water may be the easiest way of checking whether the child is able to initiate successful sucking-swallow coordination. Taste stimulation when food is applied to the child's lips or tongue may also give valuable information. When food is accepted on the lips, this might show that aversion is not present. The term "oral aversion," which frequently appears in medical studies [18] and reports, is not a distinct and independent diagnosis per se but an understandable reaction to the artificial and sometimes intrusive feeding situation, often lasting for months and involving repeated irritating and traumatizing procedures.

So identify the basic potential of the child to learn and be able to eat. Check for symptoms of tube dependency. Encourage early non-nutritive and furthermore nutritive oral stimulation if safe swallow function is present although the child is on ENT. Provide additional attention to oral feeding trials. Check for parents' ability to support their child, which may be impaired by psychiatric problems as well as unfavorable psychosocial circumstances [19].

References

1. https://journals.sagepub.com/doi/abs/10.1177/1941406409333988. Accessed 8 June 2021.
2. https://journals.sagepub.com/doi/abs/10.1177/1941406411416359. Accessed 8 June 2021.
3. Spitz RA. Hospitalism. Psychoanal Study Child. 1945;1(1):53–74. https://doi.org/10.108 0/00797308.1945.11823126.
4. https://www.youtube.com/watch?v=NelpARXhoZY, Acessed 27 April 2022.
5. Beckenbach H (2011) Developmental impact of a standardized tube weaning program (EAT: early autonomy training; Graz model for weaning tube dependency in infancy). Unpublished doctoral thesis. Medical University Graz (MUG).
6. Craig GM. Psychosocial aspects of feeding children with neurodisability. Eur J Clin Nutr. 2013;67:S17–20.
7. Craig GM, Carr LJ, Cass H, Hastings RP, Lawson M, Reilly S, Ryan M, Townsend J, Spitz L. Medical, surgical, and health outcomes of gastrostomy feeding. Dev Med Child Neurol. 2006;48(5):353–60. https://doi.org/10.1017/S0012162206000776.
8. Marinschek S, Dunitz-Scheer M, Pahsini K, Geher B, Scheer P. Weaning children off enteral nutrition by netcoaching versus onsite treatment: a comparative study. J Paediatr Child Health. 2014;50(11):902–7. https://doi.org/10.1111/jpc.12662.
9. Marinschek S, Pahsini K, Scheer PJ, Dunitz-Scheer M. Long-term outcomes of an interdisciplinary tube weaning program: a quantitative study. J Pediatr Gastroenterol Nutr. 2019;68(4):591–4. https://doi.org/10.1097/MPG.0000000000002264.
10. Kurien M, White S, Simpson G, Grant J, Sanders DS, McAlindon ME. Managing patients with gastrostomy tubes in the community: can a dedicated enteral feed dietetic service reduce hospital readmissions? Eur J Clin Nutr. 2012;66:757.

11. Jadcherla S, Khot T, Moore R, Malkar M, Gulati IK, Slaughter JL. Feeding methods at discharge predict long-term feeding and neurodevelopmental outcomes in preterm infants referred for gastrostomy evaluation. J Pediatr. 2017;181:125–30.

12. Williams C, VanDahm K, Stevens LM, Khan S, Urich J, Iurilli J, Linos E, Williams DI. Improved outcomes with an outpatient multidisciplinary intensive feeding therapy program compared with weekly feeding therapy to reduce enteral tube feeding dependence in medically complex young children. Curr Gastroenterol Rep. 2017;19(7):33. https://doi.org/10.1007/s11894-017-0569-6.

13. Sharp WG, Volkert VM, Stubbs KH, Berry RC, Clark MC, Bettermann EL, McCracken CE, Luevano C, McElhanon B, Scahill L. Intensive multidisciplinary intervention for young children with feeding tube dependence and chronic food refusal: an electronic health record review. J Pediatr. 2020;223:73–80.e2. https://doi.org/10.1016/j.jpeds.2020.04.034.

14. Stahl SM. The last diagnostic and statistical manual (DSM): replacing our symptom-based diagnoses with a brain circuit-based classification of mental illnesses. CNS Spectr. 2013;18(2):65–8. https://doi.org/10.1017/s1092852913000084.

15. Zimmerman J, Fisher M. Avoidant/restrictive food intake disorder (ARFID). Curr Probl Pediatr Adolesc Health Care. 2017;47(4):95–103. https://doi.org/10.1016/j.cppeds.2017.02.005.

16. Attia E, Becker AE, Bryant-Waugh R, Hoek HW, Kreipe RE, Marcus MD, Mitchell JE, Striegel RH, Walsh BT, Wilson GT, Wolfe BE, Wonderlich S. Feeding and eating disorders in DSM-5. Am J Psychiatr. 2013;170(11):1237–9.

17. Kuehnelt-Leddihn M, Trabi T, Dunitz-Scheer M, Burmucic K, Scheer P. Infant botulism. Causes, therapy, aftercare. Monatsschr Kinderheilk. 2009;157(9):911–3.

18. Edwards S, Davis AM, Bruce A, Mousa H, Lyman B, Cocjin J, Dean K, Ernst L, Almadhoun O, Hyman P. Caring for tube-fed children: a review of management, tube weaning, and emotional considerations. JPEN J Parenter Enteral Nutr. 2016;40(5):616–22. https://doi.org/10.1177/0148607115577449.

19. Sharp WG, Volkert VM, Scahill L, et al. A systematic review and meta- analysis of intensive multidisciplinary intervention for pediatric feeding disorders: how standard is the standard of care. J Pediatr. 2016;181:116–24.

It is not appropriate to copy the following content as a typical method of treatment. It is not a "how to do." Throughout our careers, we have taught and lectured, explained, and discussed and still find it hard or nearly impossible to outline and define the crucial details of our work. If a plan is adapted using the Graz model of tube weaning, it might work, but that's not enough. Medically fragile children are at a risk of experiencing complications of all sorts, and it is irresponsible to endanger them just by defining speed or volume of the reduction of the ENT in this chapter.

Tube weaning should not be attempted by anyone without experience and specific training. Tube weaning is invasive and needs to be respected and treated accordingly. If it fails, there is no blood, but the damage can be great or even irreversible. The following list is a summary of the typical steps involved, but each child needs an individually tailored weaning plan depending on, and adjusted to, its preexisting oral and tactile skills, sensory pattern, and underlying medical condition:

- Analyze what has been inhibiting the development of oral skills.
- Diagnose any specific oral skill deficiency or an early feeding disorder.
- Confirm tube dependence if present.
- Confirm the mutual decision to end ENT and make a plan with the parents.
- Reduce tube feeds significantly based on the child's individual growth parameter, age, underlying medical condition (especially lung, heart, and kidney function), and current medication and preexisting oral skills.
- Offer appropriate food every few hours, if possible, play picnics [1] with other children of the same age group and encourage self-determined exploration.
- Daily medical/pediatric supervision must be ensured.
- Further reduction of tube feeds should be adjusted to oral catch up and weight course.
- Tube removal and the final end of tube feeds as soon as possible and as late as necessary.

© The Author(s), under exclusive license to Springer Nature
Switzerland AG 2022
M. Dunitz-Scheer, P. J. Scheer, *Child-led Tube-management and Tube-weaning*,
https://doi.org/10.1007/978-3-031-09090-5_14

- Define a "time out" period meaning 2–3 months in which the former goal of constant weight gain is set back, and oral rehabilitation can take place.
- Ensure continuous growth checks and assign a person close to the parent's home who is responsible for keeping track of weight, nutrition, and growth.

Reviewing the literature on tube weaning [2], the common goal of all weaning efforts is the assisted and supervised discontinuation of ENS after safe, sufficient, and sustainable oral intake and age-appropriate eating practices have been established. The emerging oral skills, which compensate for the gradual reduction of ENT, can be encouraged or disturbed by intensive external stimulation, as applied in many behavioral programs. These stimulations can be behavioral psychotherapy including programs like parent counseling after every videotaped eating session, demonstrating how to feed a child by an expert (an SLT or a physiotherapist), or it may be an additional stimulation of the oral region by an SLT, but any disturbance of the child's path is potentially harmful. We ourselves have seen kids who needed a moment when the therapists from our team gave them a clear signal that they now had to leap over their resistance. An external observer can appear intrusive when feeding using a so-called finger feeder, which bypasses the lips as the first guardians of one's mouth. Looking at the situation when a finger-feeder is used, it may seem as if the child was submitted to force feeding, but looking more closely one can gain more insight and see that the child decides the frequency of the feeds and its amounts, can spit out, and is never kept closely, and all signs of resistance such as moving its head away or trying to escape the situation are respected. It's not always easy to coach parents in these moments as they may be too interested in the amount of food the child is receiving. It may be necessary to explain that the aim of the intervention is to make the child familiar with the texture and the taste of food and eventually induce a swallow reaction. This might be true for children who have never eaten by themselves because something like silent aspiration is suspected. An intervention like this should be made by parents themselves with some guidance. Never show parents that you as an expert know how to feed their baby better than them. It diminishes self-assurance and reduces competence as a caregiver, and all for the sake of a moment when the "expert" feels superior.

This is also true when following the child's personality and cues that are appropriate in its developmental state. Our data [3] on exclusive online coaching, performed by experienced tube weaning experts, reaches success rates above 90% while omitting the risk of hospital-acquired infection and offering the luxury of home-based treatment, which might be specifically indicated for immune suppressed children, those on home ventilation, or children suffering from chronic infections (like klebsiella) or psychologically traumatized patients suffering from their inpatient stay.

Following the actual start of a tube weaning project, the typical difficulties arise. It's often not only the child that is tube dependent, but also its close environment: parents, relatives, caregivers, and attending experts. Until the start of the tube weaning, the involved systems have administered precise amounts and volumes, and during the tube weaning process, this changes step by step at the child's pace, but also according to the ability and flexibility of its environment. Parents get to know their child in a completely new way and sometimes even feel like they are observing and witnessing a "new" child. The child's mood changes at first due to hunger gradually creeping in, but it is still confused and unable to identify this aversive feeling as hunger. The link between its needs and food intake has not been established yet.

In this phase the child needs to be left to find out on its own how to explore possible solutions for its new feelings. Every intervention may be counterproductive. Full protection offered by the feeding team and the parents is requested in this phase!

Well-intended remarks such as "Don't you want to try this or that" may drive the child into active resistance and opposition. The same is true for questions by parents toward the day care system such as "Has my child eaten?", "How much has the child swallowed, how much has been spilled?", "Why has the child not had a bowel movement for two days?", "Can the weight be accurate, if we weigh the stool?", "Has my child had enough to drink, or will he/she become dehydrated?", "What would happen if my child became dehydrated?", etc. These are understandable questions parents have, which come up frequently, and should be answered as part of the therapeutic dialogue. Of course, the answers differ from child to child and need to be adjusted to the individual situation.

To create appetite, it's necessary and compulsory to reduce the number of tube feeds. This must be done in a straightforward and matter of fact way and enough so that the child feels that something has changed. Different methods can be discussed, but basically it comes down to using a quick step by step approach of getting down to 40–50% of the child's original intake volume within 2–3 days. The lower limit of total fluids/kg bodyweight can and must be defined by the project leading senior pediatrician. We always proceed on an individual basis and in accordance with the child's preexisting oral skills and underlying diagnosis. We must always ensure sufficient volume, but, if the child is thoroughly full, it cannot and won't develop interest in food, neither touching it, nor licking it, and nearly never tasting food. Our research [4] has shown that the amount of enteral nutrition needs to be reduced as quickly as possible. If nutrition is reduced very slowly and hesitantly, conditions resemble those of chronic malnutrition during times of war or food shortages. The hunger-satiety system will then adjust to the reduced amount of nutrition, and one learns that there is less food available and consequently eats and needs less, but when the child experiences (for the first time) appetite due to a quick lack of ENT, it will increase its interest in food and make it possible to take further steps of self-induced food intake. Since the reduction of tube-fed nutrition requires good observation, clinical experience, and expertise, it's impossible for parents to take these steps on their own.

Often the child will start to eat unexpectedly and suddenly as if by chance. A shy and skeptical interest to touch and hold any kind of finger food might suddenly change into an intrinsic desire to lick, taste, bite, and even eat all day long. Even though the child has no idea how to chew, it does know what to do intuitively and will make huge progress in catching up with its delayed eating and drinking development depending on its motivation and the given environmental support. The child may start to demand to receive food independently, want to touch it, and even guide it to its mouth. This moment is sheer delight for anyone observing it, and at the same time, it indicates a highly delicate phase: the journey, which has just begun, will have its ups and downs, and sometimes there will also be setbacks. This is a normal developmentally driven learning in early childhood. The child will not perform and eat equally well every day; some days will be better, some worse. Also, the parents won't behave in the same way every day, and there will be days of joy and security as well as days of despair. During this process, support needs always to be available! In this initial phase, the content and distinct quality of the food and the nutritional value plays a minor role. Educational standards and ideals, such as table manners, should not matter during this phase. Food-related thoughts like "This is unhealthy" or "My child should not eat this" are not helpful at all. The child itself picks the food, and it might only be chocolate and sweets or sausages and ketchup. If ketchup is the only nutrition—we have seen once or twice that it may lead to an overload of acid—then it must be stopped quickly. If the child can eat by itself, it is also a good idea to make food available in the immediate proximity of the child for a defined period of time, day and night, so that it can decide when it can and wants to eat. The goal is to place the child in a kind of food paradise, in which it is allowed to do anything it likes following its own intentions and plans.

A transition period needs to be prepared and anticipated by the feeding team during which the child already takes and tastes food, but not in sufficient quantities to meet its full energy requirements. During this phase, the required quantity of tube nutrition must be adjusted daily depending on how much will still be necessary to support the child. The time needed from this point until all tube feeds can be stopped completely can differ widely and depends on a variety of factors, such as the progress the child makes, the anxiety of the parents, the pace in which swallowing becomes easy, and problems which are part of an underlying illness. Even if tube feeding has been stopped completely, it may be necessary, on occasion, to return to an intermediate interval of tube feeding, for example, during a flu or other illness.

This phase might be perceived as being turbulent or strenuous by parents. Therefore, it needs to be explained in advance as an expected and normal part of the weaning process. Parents tend to assume that their child will not have to undergo these problems, as they think that they themselves are not "tube dependent," meaning that they are accustomed to support their infant's life by giving it tube feds many times a day. The explanations may not be understood adequately in advance. This does create a change. Even if so, it's still better to offer them, because it might be easier to remember these explanations when necessary.

A child can be defined as being tube-weaned when it has learnt to sustain itself exclusively by oral intake for more than 35 days after the last tube feed and can feed itself or be fed orally with a stable weight, but treatment may not be finished at this point. While the child may have learnt to eat, parents can still feel insecure and lack confidence in their child's ability to eat sufficiently. It might be too early for them to be released from treatment into autonomy without additional therapeutic support. Some children also stick to just a few highly selected foods, which might be regarded as being insufficient for a healthy nutrition. Other children are unable to deal with solid foods. They encounter difficulties with lumps and may be afraid to choke even on small crumbs. Another group have special needs, and although they are able to eat, they can't be taken out in public, because they spill or soil themselves with food or display behaviors, which are socially unacceptable.

It may also be the case that the child's local medical support system is not comfortable from the beginning of the tube weaning and may be anxious about making sure that the nutritional results of the tube weaning are sufficient. Doctors may argue that the child is too slim afterward or that the ingested food is not meeting standardized requirements. These are some of many other issues that can come up after successful tube weaning. For this reason, we have developed an aftercare program which is designed to support parents during the time needed to learn that it takes time and patience to accommodate the new situation. This support is offered online and might be necessary to stabilize the progress which has been made.

14.1   Timing and Transcultural Aspects of Tube Withdrawal

The timing of the transition of enteral to oral intake is of utmost importance. Choosing to start this task too early may endanger the intended nutritional goals; however, waiting too long increases the risk of tube dependence, complications, and side effects like psychological resistance, food avoidance, and oral aversion. Risks associated with a delayed weaning process are generally higher than those linked to weaning too early. Since adult concerns and fears influence timing immensely, whether it is from a professional and/or parental side, they need to be taken seriously, analyzed closely, and seen as obstacles to a necessary weaning process for the child's development.

Time-Related Considerations *Before* Weaning Are:

- Has a safe swallow function been confirmed, or does this issue need more specific clinical re-evaluation?
- Has the nutritional goal been achieved?
- Is the parents' mindset conducive to weaning, or are they insecure, ambiguous, doubtful, or mentally dependent on the tube?
- Is the child prepared in terms of hand-motor coordination, non-nutritive oral skills, smell and taste stimulation, touching food, etc.?
- Have any medical reasons for continuation of ENS been suggested or excluded? Are any surgeries planned for the near future?
- Is the child in the best possible nutritional state? If possible, a slight increase of weight before the planned weaning is advisable. This is to prepare for the expected slight weight drop caused by the necessary reduction of tube feeds, which allow the child to experience hunger.
- Can the child "afford" the loss of 5–10% of its bodyweight, or is the ENS inefficient, presenting no benefit to weight gain anymore?
- Is there an experienced feeding team that will take over full responsibility and be available during the tube weaning phase, including the provision of medical back up for any emergency?

Tube weaning is urgent when the transition to oral feeds does not happen spontaneously after medical reasons for keeping the child on ENT are no longer present. The process of tube weaning is defined as the full transition from enteral to oral feeds. The ease of transition is dependent on the child's age (the earlier, the easier), its preexisting oral skills, readiness, ability to touch and taste foods (hand-mouth coordination), its personality, motivational state, and the ability to perform oral explorations. A safe swallow function is essential and indispensable but can rarely be assessed by fluoroscopy or swallow test. The decision whether a child can swallow safely is usually made by observations made by parents, SLTs, and MDs.

Most children tolerate tube feeding and succeed in meeting their nutritional targets, especially if they have been tube fed since birth. They learn quickly that the mouth exists only for making noises, while their food arrives via a plastic tube. They experience no taste, just a large volume of enriched formula pumped in every few hours. They possibly manage to accept some tiny traces of food on their lips, but usually any offering of oral feed is met with disinterest or refusal. On average this group of children will be tube fed for 3–6 months, and when they meet their nutritional goals, have stable lung function, and have safe swallowing, they easily switch to oral feeding assuming they have been able to preserve some basic oral activity. When oral skills are present, they undergo gradual but swift reduction of the tube feeds under medical supervision while simultaneously increasing oral intake. A child who is interested in eating without emotional hesitations or aversive sensory issues is more than happy with the tube feed reduction, which induces a feeling of appetite and advances confidently toward food, beginning with touching, holding, licking, biting, tasting, and swallowing small amounts of whatever is available within days. Children who can sit upright unaided may have reached an age of independent activity and be candidates for finger food, solids, or semi-solid food, which can be portioned out and picked by the child. Younger children will transition to blended baby food or, in some instances, to bottle-feeds. From a child's perspective, learning to eat is as natural as learning to walk. In supportive environment infants typically pick up these skills without needing any prompting or manipulation. Nevertheless, the best environment for learning to eat is in groups of children such as in nurseries and kindergartens or at children's parties. Adults are not always helpful in this process, as they make too much fuss, trying to force the child to imitate them or by maneuvering the child, risking irritation and even refusal. The best way to learn to eat as a part of the family is to have the child join in the usual mealtimes and allow additional time to explore and experiment. Most oral skills will develop with increased sufficiency and speed, the more attention is taken away from them.

A small number of children do not adjust to tube feeding with ease and seem to get very little benefit from it. These children are faced with daily traumas from being fed, and they may frequently pull out the tube, only to have it forcibly replaced (with best intentions). Feeding times become a battle between the child and caregivers, even if the child reacts with vomiting, gagging, retching, and repeated tube removal—the tube feeding goes on—a daily torture for the child and parents. The clock, calculator, and scales become dictators of a regiment consisting of power struggles, desperate to support the child's growth. Despite the emotive descriptions, no person should be blamed for this, and we always assume that everyone wants what is best for the child. What is needed is to step back, look at the problem from the outside, and find a way to break the vicious cycle. For parents, the period of tube feeding can be either a relief or a worry. When the tube feeding is successful, it is wonderful to see the child growing but it can feel unnatural to feed a child via tube. Even though the child was too immature or ill to be fed orally, parents may feel ashamed or guilty. Psychological support is crucial when parents feel as if they are drowning in negative emotions. Parents will usually start to wonder about the cessation of tube feeding, either when a child meets its treatment targets or if tube feeding becomes more and more traumatic or unsuccessful.

The less successful tube feeding is the more traumatized parents are. Pediatricians may have to suggest tube weaning after attempting a variety of ENS. Even from a medical perspective, planning discontinuation of tube feeding can be straightforward and easy, or ambivalent and conflicting. When the child has successfully met its goals, the weaning process should be started, but unfortunately, the child is obliged to switch between teams involved in fitting the tube and the aftercare. Sometimes the child can become stuck by seeing trainees, specialized nurses, or dieticians. No senior clinician is present who can decide to stop tube feeding. Concurrently, the child may be tube fed longer than necessary simply due to lack of a decision-maker being present. Tube weaning requires an interdisciplinary team favorably composed of dieticians, speech therapists (SLTs), psychologists, and pediatricians—mentioned in other chapters. It is important to have these professionals in the team and to ensure that the necessary decisions can be made in a timely manner.

Recent studies have found that up to 30% of children who are tube dependent are severely malnourished, which is a worrying result. Tube weaning teams are increasingly put together, step by step, with a variety of treatment options, including online—where the child can be weaned successfully and safely at home. Speaking as physicians to other physicians, our priority is to ask medical professionals to listen to parent's concerns surrounding all of the difficulties having to do with enteral nutrition and to consider tube weaning as a solution sooner rather than later, to avoid the pitfalls of tube dependence.

References

1. A report was published by us in Signal, the newspaper of WAIMH (World Association for Infant Mental Health): https://perspectives.waimh.org/wp-content/uploads/sites/9/2017/05/From-Each-Side-of-the-Tube.-The-Early-Autonomy-Training-EAT-Program-for-Tube-dependent-Infants-and-their-Parents.pdf. Accessed 22 August 2021.
2. Gardiner AY, Fuller DG, Vuillermin PJ. Tube-weaning infants and children: a survey of Australian and international practice. J Paediatr Child Health. 2014;50(8):626–31. https://doi.org/10.1111/jpc.12608.

3. Marinschek S, Dunitz-Scheer M, Pahsini K, Geher B, Scheer P. Weaning children off enteral nutrition by netcoaching versus onsite treatment: a comparative study. J Paediatr Child Health. 2014;50(11):902–7. https://doi.org/10.1111/jpc.12662.
4. Krasnovsky A (2004) Qualitative Therapieevaluation nach erfolgter Sondenentwöhnung bei frühkindlichen Ess- und Fütterungsstörungen. [Dissertation] Medical University Graz. https://online.medunigraz.at/mug_online/wbAbs.showThesis?pThesisNr=14733&pOrgNr=1&pPersNr=51828, Accessed 27 April 2022.

The Specific Role of the Individual Professions Within the Feeding Team

In all cases where the nutritional goal of ENT has been achieved, a weaning program should be chosen under experienced medical and therapeutic supervision. If the nutritional goal has not been achieved by ENS, a quantitative and qualitative evaluation of the ENS and the interference of other aversive factors are necessary. In cases when growth is being supported by ENS, but the intended and initially defined goals have not been achieved yet, one can wait and define a new timeframe while continuously striving to reach those goals.

Fortunately, the transition from enteral to oral feeding can occur naturally and without any specific difficulties and "by chance" without therapy. The phenomenon of spontaneous self-weaning happens more naturally and easily if ENT did not end active oral intake. If that is the case, even a child on ENT may express discrete cues indicating its emerging interest in food and beverages. In response to these cues, parents can react in a supportive way and refrain from any criticism at joint meals. This makes all the difference.

Professional interventions to wean from tube dependency must be recognized as a medical necessity in patients who don't transit to orality by themselves, and health centers as well as insurance authorities should accept tube weaning as a compulsory follow-up intervention for tube dependency after temporary tube placement.

In the case of transitioning a medically fragile child from ENT to oral feeds, close monitoring of medical, nutritional, and psychological status over the course of a few weeks is necessary to ensure the safety of the child, enable the intended reduction of enteral volumes, and support an increase in oral compensation.

The role of each participant in the weaning process depends predominantly on their personality, specific training, professional role, and knowledge about the child and its family. We will try to outline the main tasks for each professional involved. If more than one medical doctor and one member of the therapeutic team are actively involved, it is crucial to establish excellent communication and coordination

© The Author(s), under exclusive license to Springer Nature
Switzerland AG 2022
M. Dunitz-Scheer, P. J. Scheer, *Child-led Tube-management and Tube-weaning*,
https://doi.org/10.1007/978-3-031-09090-5_15

between them and the family to avoid misunderstandings and delays. The descriptions do not claim content coverage and are, of course, unavoidably influenced by the pediatric perspective.

(a) The **pediatrician** in the feeding team is responsible for the child's general medical suitability, current and ongoing medical state, and well-being before and during the weaning process. Depending on the diagnosis, it is in their discretion whether to involve additional medical experts. During the weaning process, the child's prior doctors may serve as external advisory board and for on-site evaluation when unexpected problems occur. In cases of acute illness or deterioration of the child, which may be attributed to the reduction of tube feeds, the pediatrician must change the course of action or interrupt the weaning process and possibly change the plans for weaning after recovery. The continuous availability during the weaning process is of paramount importance for both the child and its parents and will have great influence on the handling of intervening irregularities and outcomes. During aftercare, the pediatrician is responsible for the medical report, regular growth checkups, and medical advice.

(b) The **psychologist** has a very different role and responsibility. They must be well trained in developmental psychology and of course in early eating development. At the same time, the psychologist often finds her−/himself in the role of creating a bridge between parents and doctors. Other tasks include continuously keeping track and interpreting all new information, new behavior shown, and the child's hunger and satiety cues. Any additional developmental issues like toddlers' oppositional phases, and mild, moderate, to severe developmental delays, signs of autism spectrum disorder (ASD), or in fact any kind of additional psychological deviation such as trauma or anxieties, are also in the psychologist's realm of issues to deal with while assisting with tube weaning. Psychologists may have an impact on research by examining and defining the academic questions for studies and making sense the scientific outcomes.

(c) The **psychotherapist** is not an unconditional but a highly recommended complement to the composition of a feeding team. Their task is to question, interpret, and coordinate different opinions, perceptions, and perspectives belonging to everyone involved, for the sake of the child moving forward. This role functions as an advocate of the child and its perspective. The core responsibility of this person is to keep the child's emotional state and level of cognitive understanding in the center of focus. In cases where additional therapeutic support of traumatized parents is needed, or assistance with the symbolic play of the child, the role of the psychotherapist is often indispensable. We strongly advocate for child-led schools, a psychoanalytic assessment, and a strictly non-behavioral approach.

(d) Any **nurse** who has known the tube-fed child since the period of his or her tube placement is invaluable and may even override all other professional assistances during tube management and well-focused recommendations on the issue of withdrawal from tube feeds. If available this can be the smoothest and most efficient support, as their observation of the best timing for the transition to oral feeds will be early, and knowing the child and its family from the start of ENS enables more specific and individually tailored assistance. Their main job will be taking care of all physical complications, such as chronic skin irritation, dislocation, and other tube-related issues.

(e) The **dieticians/nutritionists' task** is the calculation of all required nutritional intake including vitamin, mineral, and micronutrient supplementation. During tube feeding, this is offered in the specific nutrition prepared by pharmaceutical companies. The storage is usually completely full, so worrying about supplementation should only start when a child doesn't proceed from a reduced diet (like eating only certain yoghurts or puddings) to a bigger variety of food. When the child is exclusively on enteral feeds, nutrition is calculated by a dietician. In the transition process, experienced professionals leading the weaning process risk weight loss, as well as insufficient supplementation of necessary nutritional elements. Later on, the dietician may be asked to calculate sufficient nutrition in respect to fat, protein, and carbohydrates. The task is easily defined in numbers, but its implication, acceptance, execution, and practical implementation can be challenging. Sometimes children don't gain weight even when on ENT because vomiting and poor compliance withhold the effect of ENT. In these cases, the discussion between the feeding team and a nutritionist may cause stress within the team. Our advice is to stay calm and evaluate the pros and cons of ENT. In the end, an oral nutrition seems in most cases to lead to better results than ENT with calculated food and liquid intake, which was unsuccessful for more than 4 to 6 months [1].

The ongoing discussion [2] about the benefits and disadvantages of standardized versus homemade blended food needs to be carefully supervised by a nutritionist. Homemade blended food needs supervision, because self-made enteral nutrition may lack specific items such as micronutrients or even essential fatty or amino acids. Some experts don't want to take the risk of malnutrition no matter how strongly the family argues for self-made enteral nutrition and adamantly recommend the processed food. In this debate, parents may withdraw from readily sharing their views and accepting supervision. This may lead to major deficiencies in food supply for their infant, while other side effects of enteral nutrition like vomiting may subside. A lack of essential proteins, fats, minerals, vitamins, or micronutrients may lead to insufficient thriving. When the tube-fed child receives homemade food from its parents (because of recurrent vomiting or because of the parent's convictions), the nutritionist/dietician should make prescriptions for individually tailored food. Adjustments of recommendations depending on the child's gut tolerance and the possible occurrence of GERD should be respected. Dietary limitations such as food intolerances or allergies must be acknowledged in all cases, and in children with inborn failures of metabolism, prescriptions should be made in coordination with a biochemist.

(f) The **occupational therapist** can be defined as being the main person responsible for all issues belonging to the child's sensory perception. This involves general tactile recognition and subsequently stimulation. Furthermore, an occupational therapist covers the questions of tasting, smelling, ability, intent to touch food, dealing with food soiling, etc. Attention should also be focused on mealtime routines, general sensory patterns, individual limitations like motor planning and ability to coordinate hand-mouth movements, and individual preferences. Their work is to directly address the child and includes multiple and diverse levels beyond food, such as general perception and dealing with limitations like movement insecurities and handicaps regarding hand-mouth coordination. The tools used should be colorful, attractive, and stimulating.

(g) The **physiotherapist** deals with posture and positioning. Imagining a child drinking water while lying flat on its back or bending forward helps us understand what is not possible and needs to change to function. Nevertheless, we do remember a 3-year-old boy who drank exclusively lying on its back without coughing, but after teaching him to sit upright while drinking, the amount of fluid and even nutrition swallowed increased tremendously. Any child with hypotonic muscular patterns, in general, or specifically in its trunk, neck, and head, will have difficulties in chewing and swallowing. An upright position is also a prerequisite for looking at food, wanting to touch it, and using one's hands to reach for it. The function of physiotherapy is also to observe the "bigger picture" of how sitting looks during mealtimes and offer suggestions for moving toward a situation in which the child is encouraged to take an active and independent part in the self-feed.

(h) The **speech and language therapists** are often assigned as the first therapist. They may feel responsible for the preparation of oral skills and stimulation to induce oral activity. From our perspective, the education of SLT (speech language therapists) is too centered in orality inducing, which is a therapy approach which focuses on the oral region and tries to overcome oral resistance and withdrawal of the child, who may not want to be stimulated around their traumatized oral zone. We advocate a more holistic approach, which respects the child's signals and doesn't interfere with its highly reactive parts on the face. Sometimes even unpleasant therapeutic measures are taken, such as intruding into the mouth without the child's consent. Although it might be necessary to confront a child with flavor and texture of food when trying to overcome oral resistance, an underlying respect toward its physical autonomy may lead to better results. Therefore, we oppose any force-feeding attempts by SLTs. The observations of low muscular tone and oral dysfunctions made by SLTs describe the symptoms of any child who has not used their mouth for nutritional intake for months or even since birth. This must be considered, and the SLT's advice should be valued. Many SLT professionals in our group have had additional training topics such as Castillo Morales therapy. They may advise the parents to stimulate the child's mouth, which is helpful in some cases, but it's intrusive and bears the risk of inducing stronger oral resistance. Children don't start eating just because they have received intraoral stimulation. Their motivation stems from the feeling of hunger and satiety within a safe environment, which supports their learning steps. Their social environment may motivate them to join a meal or take part in the family's meals. Starting non-nutritive stimulation performed by an SLT may be highly effective as early as in the NICU but needs to be done with utmost caution and sensitivity.

(i) The **social worker** is a very valuable member of the feeding team and helps organize family support, age-appropriate activities like day care, equipment for special needs, and the integration of the children and their families into existing social support and activities which they might not be aware of. Additional financial support or activities offered by the healthcare system may be an option that was unknown. When a tube-fed child visits day care institution, it might need additional caretakers for tube feeding during the day. In most cases the families need some additional help and assistance for managing the challenges of family life while offering ENT, especially if there are other siblings to be taken care of.

(j) **Music therapy** doesn't directly enhance oral intake but can be helpful in supporting the traumatized tube-fed child on its voyage to start trusting the world after long hospitalizations. Such children seem to have reduced their circle of trust in a way, where all adults, sometimes including close family members, make them suspicious and cautious about almost anything! Particularly in infants and very young or disabled children, the capacity for active dialogue and self-induced preverbal communication by gestures, mimics, and visual cues is a crucial prerequisite before becoming interested in the world of foods, tastes, and textures.

(k) **Hydrotherapy**, like music therapy, also serves the basic sensory and emotional core of the self, as well as many interpersonal and inter-relational issues. The water environment in a specially designed pool is probably the only treatment not involving any food, and the contact of the tube-fed child with water in combination with being held and protected by its person of attachment can help greatly to support self-confidence and later independence.

(l) **Clown:** if a team has the luxury of being able to receive the support of a trained hospital clown to visit children and make them happy and laugh, it is one of the very best components of a positive treatment environment! The process of learning to eat does not only demand attention to the actual and immediate steps of oral functions and skills but also needs a lot of new motivation and ease, and any activity diverting stress and hardship from the child is welcome. In addition to a very general effect clowns have on children, they are specially trained in communication and interactive dialogues and can engage with the child on an encouraging and joyful level to try new things.

References

1. Khan Z, Marinschek S, Pahsini K, Scheer P, Morris N, Urlesberger B, Dunitz-Scheer M. Nutritional/growth status in a large cohort of medically fragile children receiving long-term Enteeral nutrition support. J Pediatr Gastroenterol Nutr. 2016;62(1):157–60. https://doi.org/10.1097/MPG.0000000000000931.
2. Koletzko S. Progress of enteral feeding practice over time: moving from energy supply to patient- and disease-adapted formulations. Nestle Nutr Workshop Ser Pediatr Program. 2010;66:41–54. https://doi.org/10.1159/000318947.

16

Hospitals in general are not built or intended to be equipped for providing surroundings that promote developmental processes. Developmentally based learning rarely takes place in an environment associated with fear, anxiety, and interventions experienced as traumas, often creating memories of painful moments. Hospitals must be sterile, smelling of cleaning fluids, and not of cooked food. The staff usually does not encourage children to comfortably make a mess in the process of learning to eat, which is a helpful tool while learning. Currently almost all hospitals serve food which was prepared in a kitchen far away from the patient and does not have the flexibility to change anything about the food if the child is disgusted by it. Prior to this way of serving food, we had tiny kitchens in wards where different finger food was stored and little dishes could be prepared. When food was given to children and even adults, patients could choose from a variety of dishes displayed on a cart, kept warm by steam. All this was taken away due to hygiene regulations, which shed a light on what is important in a hospital. The aim of a hospital is to repair illness and restore health. Eating is not part of regaining one's health, because this can be done after discharge.

We believe that an infant learning to eat needs the freedom to spill and to experiment, nudge, and spit. This is especially apparent when infants learn to eat after natural development was not possible, and they need even more freedom to learn. An encouraging environment is a key component to make progress, and restrictive rules are not.

It is an important reminder to note that hospitals smell of cleaning fluids and detergents and not of food like in restaurants, because for appetite, interest, and pleasure regarding food to change toward oral food, the child and parents' mindset needs to change with the support of the team working in the ward. The only reason to choose a hospital-based venue for tube weaning would be because of a trained and experienced feeding team and the option of monitoring breath and/or blood counts, if necessary, from a medical perspective.

M. Dunitz-Scheer, P. J. Scheer, *Child-led Tube-management and Tube-weaning*, https://doi.org/10.1007/978-3-031-09090-5_16

There are efficient alternatives to plan a tube weaning process outside of the hospital setting:

- Online counseling introduced years ago, applying the "Netcoaching [1]" model successfully in cooperation with a local medical backup.
- Using an Eating-School venue, which is a project we started in Graz. It is specifically designed and equipped for the transition to orality in children. The age of the referred children varies between 6 months and young adolescence. The venue contains everything needed for tube weaning, for example, a cook, a team that works mainly "undercover" and engages all the children to play with food, and special groups in which kids can, e.g., build cars and aero planes using edible items, and parents are instructed on recognition and awareness of food and food refusal. Children and their families, including siblings, are welcome.
- An outpatient approach with visits in the hospital for specific therapeutic sessions and medical checkups 2–3 times a week when frequent lab checkups might be necessary.
- A mainly home-based program with visits by members of the feeding team, including accompanying professionals that are needed.

As we are still (2022) active in counseling pediatric institutions on various aspects of making eating a more attractive experience, we have become more and more convinced that a positive eating experience doesn't happen with ease at a hospital. Aside from the benefits of laboratory surveillance, an infection may happen due to nosocomial germs. Even in adolescents suffering from severe anorexia nervosa, the best any medical center can do regarding food issues is to ensure sufficient intake (be it by means of tube feeds) and prevent further malnutrition and wasting. Evidence shows that compulsory treatment is not always effective in the long run [2]. Even patients on ENT often lose weight, and experienced centers treating anorexia nervosa are admitting that weight stabilization or gain on ENT sometimes doesn't occur. We assume that in this setting, joyful experiences are mostly restricted to therapy sessions with the speech therapists, who may offer new tastes and smells. We practiced psychosomatic therapy in a pediatric hospital for 36 years, developing a proficient and creative multidisciplinary team. Our experience and findings were the basis of a spin-off nonprofit commercial firm, which still consists of some of our former coworkers, such as the physiotherapist Eva Kerschischnik and the two clinical psychologists Sabine Marinschek and Karoline Pahsini. When we left the hospital a great deal of success in developing the tube weaning method, and built up the so-called Graz model, we founded "Notube," which offers a variety of treatment options.

There are four therapeutic settings we use/have used, which are described in detail below:

- A solely *online approach*, which we have introduced and developed for years, and defined as "Netcoaching." It is highly effective and was an innovative use of tele-health. This model is very successful [1] in tube weaning and is one of the applications we offer in addition to online counseling of adolescents suffering from anorexia nervosa and pre- and post-counseling of families taking part in the Eating-School setting. Its practical implementation includes time management and cooperation with the local medical backup. The main advantage is that the family and child can stay at home. Any meeting of the MFC on ENT with other children can be avoided. Additionally, no hospital is visited. The process of learning to eat happens in a discrete and undercover way, and when one is lucky, the child hardly even notices the achievements it has made during the transition from enteral to oral feeding. Online weaning demands confident parents who trust the therapists and medical backup, who are willing to assist in moments of insecurity, or if an acute illness demands an interruption of the program.

- *Eating-School* (ES): this is a new innovative venue, specifically designed and equipped for the needs of children and their families including siblings. Our venue is on the ground floor of a villa built in fin de siècle style. We try to be attractive and inviting to families in our quest to lead them into the world of tastes, textures, and smells of different foods on all sensory levels. The intensive "oral rehab" lasts for 12 days from 9 am to 6 pm, including three play picnics every day and many parent-child groups focusing on sensory experiences, individually tailored to every child. Medical supervision and psychological support are always at hand, and in cases of unexpected medical emergencies, the university hospital is within walking distance. The intensive hours spent in the venue and the child-led approach are specific to our ES model, and aftercare is available online. The ES program is highly effective.

- An *outpatient setting*, including visits to a hospital for therapeutic meetings and medical checkups 2–3 times/week if necessary. This is not a specifical program Notube offers currently but could be adapted if the facilities cooperate and the medical situation of a child (e.g., severe renal insufficiency) demands close lab monitoring. This model can offer various levels of intensity starting at visits only from the feeding team. Additionally specific therapeutic sessions like hydrotherapy, music therapy, sensory stimulation, speech therapy, dietary counseling, and psychological support may be offered. It allows children to continue with their usual daily routine. It needs supervision and instruction to promote an awareness of possible behavioral changes, which are expected during the planned phases of changing the tube feeding routine. We used this model in various hospitals in Israel and installed it in the large Sheba hospital on a regular basis as we had formerly developed the option in the psychosomatic outpatient clinic at the pediatric hospital in Graz. Patients were coming from the catchment areas of Styria, Burgenland, and Carinthia but rarely from Vienna. Weighing, collecting intake data, and advising further steps were helpful for a lot of families.

- A mainly *home-based* program: this model had been predominantly developed in Germany by our former student Markus Wilken. In recent years he has shifted his focus toward trauma theory in assessment and therapy. It consists of 1-week-lasting visits to the families in their homes and instructing them on the how-to-dos in the weaning process [3]. After a phase of getting to know each other, he comes into the family house and offers hands on therapies. These therapies demand the coordination of all participants of the local as well as incoming feeding team and the availability of a pediatrician offering visits either at a doctor's office or a home visit to ensure the child is in a safe medical state during the weaning experience. As there are no group activities involved, the possibility of an infection is diminished. Sometimes the duration of the transition process can last longer, but this model can be suitable for children unable to travel or forbidden to meet with other children, for example, because of immune system suppression.

Each of these methods is variations of our basic theoretical concept. They can be planned and performed in various manners or a combination of the described venues and programs. We advise to seek the most appropriate model for oneself and that the parents have the most say in the decision process, as they need to feel secure and safe to start the voyage of increasing feeding skills and become empowered to let the child move.

16.1   What Is a Play Picnic (PP)?

As a mother and father and grandmother and grandfather of a large family, we have learned that a good and joyful meal together is one of the most rewarding social interactions imaginable and needs well prepared and tasty food, but foremost, a good atmosphere. The best food cannot be enjoyable if stress or disharmony is in the air. The invention of play picnics is based on "normal family meals" and including the youngest family members. Our experience comes from the home visits and drop-in groups we were a part of during our psychotherapy training and later in our work as pediatricians running a 14-bed ward, an outpatient clinic, and as management trainers at various institutions in DACH countries.

Young and smart children who have been through many hospitalizations are justifiably suspicious, anxious, or overtly traumatized. They don't trust any adult they can't identify as being part of their circle of trust, which may be restricted to their family and no one else. On the other hand, we noticed that young children hardly ever show a defensive and fearful attitude toward other children. We became aware of how intensely children watch and playfully imitate each other. They mostly find it easier to integrate and eat with a group of children than being with only their parents. In Austria, group dynamics and group psychotherapy have a long tradition and are integrated in child-associated systems, early education (kindergartens, schools), business, and recreational institutions run by social security. Having been in multiple group therapies involving adults with and without communicational deficits and large groups integrating children of all age groups, we felt that "group therapy [4]" (according to the proposals made by Irvin Yalom in his early years before he became a bestselling author [5]) could work for babies and infants as well without communicating verbally.

The first play picnics were started in 1986 at the psychosomatic unit of the University Children's Hospital in Graz. Subsequently, we taught the indication, the strategy, and the effect of it to many experts elsewhere [6]. The structural integration of this new therapy required no additional budget, but intensive discussions with the food preparation and cleaning team, as well as the therapists involved. The food preparation had to convince the infant that it was accessible on its own. The decoration of plates, colors, and smells needed to be adapted. It shouldn't remind a child or an adult of the smell of a hospital disinfectant nor should the presentation of the food be too clean and too proper. Children needed to be able to help themselves and spilling, dropping something, and smearing yoghurt on the parent's lap was allowed. This caused problems with the cleaning team as we performed our play picnic on a wooden floor and some of the milky stuff went in the parquet floor. Additionally, they had their lunch break when we were done by 1 pm, so it took some time for the cleaning team to get enthusiastic about how to help the infants by having their room cleaned after the play picnic. The "new" smell was constantly in the room when team meetings were held, or seminars were given. Finally, therapists didn't know how to behave; should they get involved in interactions of every family member, or should they supervise the group situation and try to create a positive atmosphere? How much attention is needed? The answer is easy: you can't tell. Sometimes if a parent is starting to force-feed its child, an instant intervention is needed. This might be true also for depressed parents who are not involved at all and sit behind their child not interacting. Very agile infants sometimes steal food from everywhere, barely eating it. They are like wolves and the fun of stealing is enough for them. These children must be restricted to their "region," and parents need to take responsibility for their child. A lot of funny, demanding, and sometimes unsolvable situations arose, which needed attention.

Having a large one-way mirror for teaching and coaching, we looked at the picnic with one of the parents from behind the screen while the other one was "on the floor" with the child. A few rules [7] were installed:

1. The children have absolute priority; they may do anything and everything except for hurting or endangering themselves or others. They are the center. In the beginning it's enough that the child tolerates being in the room and feeling safe.
2. The goal is interaction and fun with food and not actually eating food. If any food is eaten, it's also fine.
3. The children are only comforted if they cry. A screaming child does not need to stay in the room. Any disruptive behavior toward others is avoided.
4. Parents must keep at a secure distance; it is best if they are seated behind their child and interfere as little as possible. Help is only offered when asked for.
5. Parents are given written information and informed about the PP rules.
6. Any professionals should be integrated as smoothly as possible and only observe but also interfere when a parent is behaving intrusively or stressfully.
7. The quantitative key is one parent per child; siblings should be encouraged to attend and no more than one professional for two children.
8. Appropriate food needs to be ordered or brought along; parents and siblings are encouraged to eat too.

16.2   Why Force Feeding Is Not an Option and Definitely Not a Solution

Feeding is vulnerable to pressure. A quick online search using Google shows 1.320.000.000 hits in 0.74 s, which tells parents how to feed their children. Sometimes even strangers on the street offer an opinion on how to get a screaming or refusing child to eat. Parents of children with an NG tube experience a roller-coaster of unwanted advice and unhelpful recommendations inducing feelings of insufficiency. When the medical team decides that feeding by tube is no longer necessary, they try to feed their child orally, but when the child shows no interest in eating, or even starts gagging and vomiting, parents and children get stressed around food and the problem starts.

As professionals who deal with tube weaning in a wide variety of conditions, we try to understand the feelings of parents whose child won't eat. Comparing one's child to the others who seem to happily be munching away on anything that is placed in front of them is difficult.

The current recommendation for healthy infants is to begin with solid food at the age of 4 to 6 months [8]. Even in children without ENS, this may be a big, sometimes unresolvable step.

The first thing to remember is that 6 months is a guideline. Some children will be ready earlier and some later. When weaning from the tube, some weight loss is to be expected, and initially, contact with food should be about exposure to new flavors and textures, without worrying too much about volume.

Some parents are lucky enough to have children, who sit like a baby bird, mouth open, and ready to accept any food given to them. However, many other children are not so easy, especially if they have been fed through a feeding tube.

If a child is spoon feeding, one may be tempted to try a little subterfuge here, by making the child laugh and sneaking in a mouthful or distract them with a toy and do the same. This process, while it gets food into them, is a short-term solution, which, in the long run, the child will learn to work around. As an adult you would also be unlikely to enjoy food that was shoved into your mouth unexpectedly when you were not hungry.

Instead, we recommend allowing the child to feed him- or herself, if possible. There are lots of finger foods that can be safely enjoyed by a 6-month-old. Just place it in front of them for them to see and touch, making sure food is available frequently to offer when the child is likely to be hungry, rather than at adult predetermined mealtimes.

If the child is a little older, one may be tempted to coax them into eating, offering a reward for trying some food or a promise of pudding, if they eat some vegetables. We want children to eat in response to hunger, rather than a desire to please their parents or get a reward. If you have tried this, you may have noticed that it rarely works. The child's desire to avoid eating is stronger than their desire for a reward and you both end up just getting frustrated. Puddings at mealtimes can be a hazardous topic, and you may feel judged by other parents, regarding what type of food is best for your child. At this point, do not worry about whether food is "healthy" or not. First, your child is likely to have a small appetite, so foods that are high in calories but small in volume are ideal. Secondly, the important thing is for your child to eat anything. A lot of children who struggle to eat are more sensitive to certain flavors and textures; this often eases as they get older, but only offering them food, which is unpleasant to them, will not encourage them to want to eat.

Parents and caregivers can easily fall into the trap of believing that refusal to eat is a matter of discipline. They might be threatening to withhold treats, unless a meal is eaten, or refusing to let the meal end, until a certain amount of food is ingested. It can often seem like the more effort you put into a meal, the more likely it is to be refused! This is where, hard though it is, one needs to step back. A child with aversion to food is not refusing it to spite you. You are not a bad parent, if you let your child turn down a meal. A child who has to force down a cold, congealed meal, while crying and gagging, is not likely to look forward to the next offering. Another temptation is to distract an older child with television or games and spoon feeding them while distracted. Although this doesn't usually distress the child, and we understand the need to have an easy meal every now and then, we don't encourage doing this very often.

When one works with parents during the tube weaning process, some of the most significant stresses for them comes from perceived and real outside judgment, i.e., the feeling that society judges' parents based on what their children eat, as well as pressure from well-meaning friends and relatives.

16.3   Do Siblings of Tube-Fed Children Suffer?

Little is known about this. "Tube-fed children" are not just tube fed. They were often born prematurely, having many stays in the hospital, and their parents were just as affected and spent a lot of time in the hospital with them. Therefore, since the birth of their tube-fed child, the parents have had to depend on outside support for the care of the sibling or siblings. If a grandmother or an aunt/uncle provided support, then the sibling wasn't so alone and can normally bridge the gap well. It is not good when the parents are alone in a strange town without any support. The mother and father of both children share many tasks, jobs and hospital stays, and they also want to give the healthy child a normal life. It is very often the case that the healthy sibling, whether older or younger, is expected to be considerate toward the sick tube-fed child. The brave sibling is considerate, but only by suppressing their own needs.

In her 1979 book *The Drama of the Gifted Child: The Search for the True Self*, Alice Miller presents a child that took the needs of adults into too much consideration. More consideration than was good for him. The child hardly thought of himself. This way of thinking often persists throughout their lives, where the others come first, and they are last. Daily life becomes self-sacrificing, putting their own needs last becomes the rule, and only when this person is seriously hurt are they able to defend themselves. This dynamic can also occur with the siblings of tube-fed children. They have to respect their needs, but this is easier said than done. The healthy child can't be considered as much as the tube-dependent child. For the healthy sibling, it is an especially difficult situation when the tube-fed child comes home from hospital and the parents are responsible for additional care duties. Even with very good care through home care nurses, for example, for children on respirators at home, the mother is always preoccupied with the care of the tube-fed child. Having more than one child can feel like a constant juggling act. From school drop-offs to nappy changes, helping with homework and cooking dinner, some days it makes you wish you had an extra pair of arms and ears or a clone or two to help.

When you have your first child, you have the time to really enjoy your baby. Snuggled in the fuzzy warmth of newborn hormones you can let the world carry on without you as you gaze lovingly at your little one and note every feature and development. Then along comes children two, three, four, or more and suddenly it's very different. The world has changed into a whirling, blurring, cycle of nagging, cooking, cleaning, and answering endless calls for assistance before collapsing into bed in exhaustion, only to start again the next morning at some unreasonable hour (and that's if you're fortunate enough not to have been woken by nocturnal demands). One of the hardest emotions to deal with when you have multiple children is the worry that they are not getting enough of your attention and that your time is taken up by doing chores instead of spending quality time with them. This can be even worse if you have a child with medical problems. Your life during the last few months has been full of hospital visits, your time taken up with managing feeds and tube care, meals eaten hurriedly in hospital canteens, home chores reduced to the bare minimum needed to keep going, not to mention the chaos that ensues when a tube gets blocked or dislodged. Your children are given out to any willing relative or friend, while you make another journey to the hospital ward for treatment. It takes effort on the part of you, your partner, and family to help keep all the children feeling loved and cared for and it's a hard time for the siblings of a child with medical needs, as they can often feel overlooked and be envious of the time their sibling gets with you during feeds and medical treatments.

One of the biggest advantages of our Netcoaching program is that you can do it in your own home. Rather than a lengthy admission where you are separated from your family, this enables you to wean at home, and you can still send your children off to school, tuck them into bed, and be there for them when they need you (which, let's face it, is all the time—especially the minute you go to the bathroom or sit down with a warm drink). It is far less disruptive than the repeated travels to the hospital, as you can contact our team from the comfort of your home using our online system, saving yourself the organizational stress and expense of travel and arranging childcare.

It can be beneficial for the child to have its siblings and routine around when you go through the weaning process. How many times have you lovingly coached and encouraged a child to learn a new skill with little success, only for them to master it in minutes when they see their peers doing it? Having regular family mealtimes where you all eat together can really help the progress. Your children can join in the play picnics, giving the child being weaned a chance to watch them and join in when they feel comfortable. Without directly encouraging the child, they can demonstrate fun activities, and by all being seated at the table for mealtimes, they can help encourage meals to become no-hassle routine behavior.

We want to help get you to the point where your family can enjoy relaxed, happy mealtimes where everyone can feel included, to be able to eat out in restaurants without your child feeling left out, to help keep the peace between your children, and, finally, to get rid of all the tube feeding paraphernalia and hassle associated with tube feeding and help all your children feel equal.

References

1. Marinschek S, Dunitz-Scheer M, Pahsini K, Geher B, Scheer P. Weaning children off enteral nutrition by netcoaching versus onsite treatment: a comparative study. J Paediatr Child Health. 2014;50(11):902–7. https://doi.org/10.1111/jpc.12662.
2. Elzakkers IF, Danner UN, Hoek HW, Schmidt U, van Elburg AA. Compulsory treatment in anorexia nervosa: a review. Int J Eat Disord. 2014;47(8):845–52. https://doi.org/10.1002/eat.22330.
3. Wilken M, Cremer V, Berry J, Bartmann P. Rapid home-based weaning of small children with feeding tube dependency: positive effects on feeding behaviour without deceleration of growth. Arch Dis Child. 2013;98(11):856–61. https://doi.org/10.1136/archdischild-2012-303558.
4. Armstrong HA. Evaluation of the parent group experience. What helps and what hinders. Int J Adolesc Med Health. 2003;15(1):31–7. https://doi.org/10.1515/ijamh.2003.15.1.31.
5. https://www.yalom.com/theory-and-practice-encounter-groups. Accessed 24 August 2021.
6. Shalem T, Fradkin A, Dunitz-Scheer M, Sadeh-Kon T, Goz-Gulik T, Fishler Y, Weiss B. Gastrostomy tube weaning and treatment of severe selective eating in childhood: experience in Israel using an intensive three week program. Isr Med Assoc J. 2016;18(6):331–5.
7. http://www.ruralhealth.org.au/12nrhc/wp-content/uploads/2013/06/Moores-Kirralee_Sandford-Debra_ppr.pdf. Accessed 24 August 2021.
8. Fewtrell M, Bronsky J, Campoy C, Domellöf M, Embleton N, Fidler Mis N, Hojsak I, Hulst JM, Indrio F, Lapillonne A, Molgaard C. Complementary feeding: a position paper by the European Society for Paediatric Gastroenterology, hepatology, and nutrition (ESPGHAN) committee on nutrition. J Pediatr Gastroenterol Nutr. 2017 Jan;64(1):119–32. https://doi.org/10.1097/MPG.0000000000001454.

17.1 Fear of Weight Loss

Fear of weight loss is the main argument of parents against the idea of tube weaning. From a medical point of view, weight loss should not exceed 10% of the initial body weight during the transition to oral eating and should be regained in 2–3 months following the weaning process. When enteral-fed infants are slightly overweight, the weight loss might have positive effects on their motor development and self-help skills. The aspect of tube weaning which is most frequently discussed is the reduction of tube feeds. Should the amount of nutrition be reduced, and if so, how much and how fast? Myths around this issue range from "the child will suffer severely" to "further development will leap forward and be compromised" or even "there might be life-long consequential damages due to malnutrition." Statements from professionals, such as these, lead to doubts and concerns in already burdened parents and may hinder the possible and necessary transition from enteral to oral nutrition. We have a clear standpoint: quick reduction of tube feeds is a prerequisite of tube weaning. All other methods lack efficiency and efficacy, and without the discomfort the child encounters due to hunger and the inner transition from an unspecific feeling of discomfort to the enlightened one that is desire, eating cannot be the answer. If a child does not want to eat, then no orality will occur. Some of our colleagues try to perform tube weaning by only counseling the parents without changing the amount of tube feds, which often ends with bad results. Some offer tube weaning as part of a rehabilitation program created for eating disorders in infancy and offer cognitive-behavioral treatment to parents, and therapists attend family meals to observe behavioral changes (what our colleagues in the Eating-School do as well, but the child is hungry due to a swift reduction of ENT). When the child lacks hunger, the family ends up being subtly or sometimes even openly blamed, an example of this is when some

M. Dunitz-Scheer, P. J. Scheer, *Child-led Tube-management and Tube-weaning*,
https://doi.org/10.1007/978-3-031-09090-5_17

feeding teams have an SLT as a main person and therapy tries to convince a fully fed and saturated child to get interest in licking, tasting, biting, and swallowing food—eventually making the parents responsible for the unsatisfactory results. We want to stress that a weight loss above 10% of the weight before tube weaning must be an indicator for re-evaluation of possible underlying illnesses, the state, and development of the child. Therefore, our method uses a swift reduction within the first week of treatment, sometimes even in the first days. Hunger will only evolve if the reduction is fast; otherwise the child adapts to less food without getting enough discomfort. Additionally, we advise parents not to carry and cuddle their crying child too much, when hunger is the reason for the child being unsettled; the cognition process of interpreting unknown discomfort as hunger should not be impeded by any distraction other than food.

17.2   Existing or Non-existing Pro-nutritive Behavior and Feeding Skills

Please observe and watch the child's behavior carefully! Do not accept narratives belonging to the observations of others; particularly parent's observations cannot be used alone. The way parents look at their child is and must be different, compared to a physician's or experts' evaluation. The advantages of an expert's view are more knowledge and less emotional involvement and no innate obligation to support and protect one's offspring. As little as 1–3 can be valuable. It provides an insight into the first symptoms of emerging feeding skills: interest in food, beginning of oral skills (babbling, sucking, licking, tasting), and motivation to eat. Feeding skills develop step by step, and oral stimulation with real food or toy foods can help, but should be supervised, because foods like apples and carrots may lead to choking. Therefore, we prefer to prepare food like chips and sweets when we encounter the child and family. It shows us hand-mouth coordination and the child's state of interest. Siblings are often present and start eating as well, which makes it possible to look at larger-scale situations, where the patient presents itself as either an eating or a resisting child.

A French family consisting of four children recently entered our clinic. All three sisters, 13, 11, and 9 years old, started immediately eating the salty chips and Haribo gummy bears that were on the little table. Only the son, who was 18 months old, wasn't interested in the displayed snacks. We learned a lot in that few minute encounter. Firstly, that the boy was the desired child, as we say in Styria: "The wish for a boy belongs to the father of many girls!"; secondly, we saw parents and siblings trying to get the boy to become interested in food; and lastly, he tried a piece of a chip to comfort his parents showing that he could lick, chew, and swallow. All these observations took only a few moments and made it possible to compose an effective treatment plan, which was based on safe swallowing and considered the over involvement of the female members of the family as a central component.

17.3 Emergence of Hunger

Tube weaning is not possible without the presence of hunger! Therefore, it is necessary to reduce feeding volumes swiftly in a controlled and medically supervised environment. No satiated child will show oral activities! It is unsafe and not recommended to wean a child without medical supervision, especially medically fragile children, who often react very critically to the change in feeding routines and may need a doctor. Most tube-fed children will not just start to eat and drink on their own, and even after reducing ENT by 30%, it may take time for the infant to recognize the new feeling as hunger. Children will not learn to eat because it is expected of them, but only due to self-motivation and an increase of feeding skills. Constant offering of food or intrusive feeding is not the right strategy and will not be successful. The critical phase of tube weaning happens on the third or fourth day: the child does not feel well, is fussy, or weeps more than usual. Parents react appropriately and try to comfort their child by cuddling and offering them food, but both understandable reactions should be minimized. Parents can inspire the child's awareness by eating themselves and without offering or presenting food. Intrusive measures like force feeding raise resistance in the child and are counterproductive for the process. In our play picnics, we create a situation in which the child can play with food, touch it, and interact with the other children. Parents tend to calculate what and how much their child has eaten during the therapeutic session, and in the beginning they are only interested in quantities and caloric intake. To understand the process in which the child is entangled takes time for the whole family. Support can be given using short interventions like changing the posture of a handicapped child or continuously asking parents to eat, because they are the role models for their infant.

Feeling hunger is a precondition for learning to eat! Based on decades of experience with hundreds of tube-fed children, we can confidently say that without hunger, nothing will work. Imagine you are served a giant ice cream sundae (with cream!) after a six-course menu. Your enthusiasm to eat it would likely be close to none. That is how fully tube-fed children feel when food is presented to them, and their experience of extreme fullness causes refusal with vomiting as a common last resort. To take an interest in eating, it is necessary that a child is hungry, which is a natural result of the swift reduction of tube feeds.

17.3.1 Feeling Hunger Does Not Indicate Starvation!

This is a crucial aspect of this debate. A child needs to feel and recognize hunger and learn how to respond to it, but the child should not suffer or be in pain, and their medical state should not be endangered! Therefore, the reduction of tube feeding must be supervised and closely monitored by professionals to guarantee basic caloric requirements and hydration of the child.

17.3.2 The Tube Feeding Reduction Must Be Supervised by Experts!

Reduction of tube feeds by people who are not specifically trained in this field can be dangerous and, in the worst cases, even lead to severe health deterioration requiring medical treatment. Uninformed but not entirely uncommon attitudes, such as "If we remove the tube, the child will start eating at some point," may also have severe and dangerous consequences. (It is comparable to the swimming lessons where trainers used to expose their pupils to deep water assuming that the wish to survive will teach them to swim. Severe traumas are recalled by people having been subject to such a dreadful lesson.) Reduction of tube feeds is a highly specialized procedure that must be tailored to each child's individual needs—based on different variables, such as medical history, growth, and oral development.

17.3.3 A Child Must Be Allowed to Experience "Messy Play" with Food While It Is Hungry!

Children who are learning to eat are like newborns in their eating development, regardless of their actual age. Frequent small meals and ongoing exposure to food and textures that are easy to handle are important. Smelling, tasting, and playing with food is a completely different experience for a hungry child compared to one whose stomach is completely full!

17.3.4 Tube Feeding Reduction Cannot Be Compensated Immediately by Oral Eating!

A child who has been tube fed for months or even years must catch up on its eating development. This can't happen within hours, days, or weeks. It takes time for a child to increase its oral intake sufficiently and to compensate the tube feeds. It is important to note that a temporary reduction of nutrition does not lead to developmental impairment. Of course, sufficient nutrition is important for growth and development in the long term, but a temporary reduction of nutrition does not compromise development. On the contrary, Hannes Beckenbach [1] a former PhD student of ours (and these days our son-in-law) was able to show that children make significant developmental progress after weaning in their social interactions, motor development, and speech.

17.4 "Unhealthy" Food Is Important and Allowed During Tube Weaning!

Learning to eat involves physiological changes and psychological efforts. It is often strenuous for children, from a motivational and technical point of view, to eat big meals after their oral region hasn't been used for eating for a long time. Therefore, it may be helpful to offer high-caloric food in small volumes. Calorically "empty" food such as vegetables, even if considered as "healthy," are not at all ideal during this phase. Of course, a transition to a balanced diet should be made later when eating skills are stable, but for the first phase of the learning-to-eat process, it is important to offer attractive, high-calorie foods such as chocolate spreads, fatty sausages, or drops and intensively tasting sweets like edible paper, which is made from starch and sugar.

These are all important factors that should be considered during a tube wean. The long-term goals of tube weaning are age and developmentally appropriate oral nutrition and adequate growth of the child. Some weight loss is to be expected during the early phase of tube feed reduction, while the child is increasing its oral activity. It is important to understand that the entire weaning process takes place over the course of months following the initial reduction of tube feeds. There should be ample time for the process, to learn eating and swallowing skills, and to achieve the long-term goals. We ask physicians as well as parents to please stay patient and be proud of the child, because every step they take is a big achievement.

The shift from a highly structured tube feeding schedule to one where the child regulates its own intake of food based on its motivation and appetite is stressful. All family members as well as the doctors must adapt. During this transition, a feeding team is needed as a prerequisite before planning treatment at an institution offering tube weaning.

Temporary weight loss is unavoidable during the weaning process; therefore, the weight course, as well as the increase and possible normalization of eating practices, must be supervised carefully before, during, and for 1 year after the tube weaning procedure has been completed. Depending on the child's weight at the onset of weaning, weight loss should not exceed 10% of body weight. A study done by our colleague Zarah Khan et al. [2] showed that more than 30% of a large, unselected population of MFCs on ENT were severely malnourished when presented for weaning after months or years of exclusive tube feeding. The reason for malnutrition was limited individual volume tolerance resulting in recurrent vomiting, hypersensitive children not being able to follow prescriptions, and wrong nutritional calculations. While some of the children on ENT are clearly overfed, some will arrive for weaning being malnourished. A malnourished child coming for weaning presents a challenge, as weight loss can't be tolerated as easily as in normal or overweight children. Additionally, from a physiological point of view, if there is almost no lipolysis, then only very few ketones are available, which are a source of appetite stimulation. Lean children at the beginning of reduction of ENT may not react to the lack of calories, and these children shouldn't be exposed to reduction for the sake of inducing appetite, but the volumes of feeds must be reduced so that side effects of ENT diminish, especially vomiting, which is a frequent problem of lean MFCs on ENT. Cessation of vomiting might already induce interest in food, stimulating eating behavior by taking part in play picnics, and family meals may also prove to be helpful.

The intervention of tube weaning must be planned and performed in a clear and detailed manner, and reducing tube feeds should not resemble an everyday routine. This would lead to a child adapting to less food and result in weight loss, lack of energy, and no eating behavior, motivation, or appetite and might harm the child. The reduction of the child's ENS can be performed quickly (transition from exclusive ENT to full oral intake in 2–3 weeks) or slowly (the same process of transition needing up to 1 year), but however scarce the literature [3] on this topic might be, it shows significant advantages of "fast weaning" [4].

Davis AM et al. [5] reported the use of a megestrol medication for tube weaning in a small sample of tube-fed infants. Another group tried medications such as antidepressants known for their appetite stimulating side effects. Results should be viewed critically because the advantages of medication to support tube weaning were little [6].

In the cases where tube weaning is clearly indicated but no experienced local therapeutic resources are available to perform weaning—or where the child is unable to be admitted into institutional care because of immune deficits—telemedicine proves to be a welcomed and highly effective alternative [7]. It offers medically supervised intensive nutritional and behavioral parent coaching, video analysis, as well as being able to involve the child's local medical and therapeutic team.

The choice of any weaning strategy is therefore dependent on the underlying medical diagnosis, its implications on appetite regulation and preexisting oral skills, and the availability of individualized therapeutic support programs with a full hospital backup. The need for laboratory tests must be planned critically and in advance, and the necessity of careful assessment, a preparation phase, an intensive tube feed reduction phase, and aftercare of sufficient duration are common to all weaning efforts.

17.5   The Role of the Parents: Supportive Versus Counterproductive

All parents love their children. In the rare cases that don't resemble the expected human relationships, the seemingly "unloving" parent is usually in serious personal trouble, either socially, emotionally, or both. Most parents and close caretakers love unconditionally, but this is manifested in individual and culturally different ways, resulting in some meeting expectations better than others.

What is special about parents of tube-fed children? When parents have not been able to feed their child in a natural way following their intuitive parenting skills [8], as the Papouseks said, normal attachment behavior doesn't evolve as easily as it should. Parents attempt to learn to suppress their natural wish to feed their baby, which is basically impossible and unnatural. To renounce this for the sake of well-justified medical arguments does not make it easier. This might explain why parents who have been informed by doctors using the most sophisticated academic explanations with the best intentions about all necessary interventions have no questions for the employees of the NICU, PICU, or surgical team other than when they will be allowed to feed their child. Professionals sometimes meet this question with confusion and lack of understanding because they feel that the parents need to shift their priorities and focus on the lifesaving effort they are making. Looking at it from a psychodynamic perspective, the moment where a parent is able to feed their child is the only thing they feel urgency about. What we mean by psychodynamic here is that there is a drive, even instinct, that leads to the irresistible wish to feed one's child. Professionals tend to define if the parents' behavior is supportive from their perspective, and they want parents to aid them in their quest and various lifesaving measures, which to them is the only behavior they recognize as adequate. Parents of medically fragile patients who have been through months of intensive care are traumatized in various degrees and are hanging by a thread on an emotional level, so professionals need to learn to modify their expectations and to observe what parents actually do, in order to make small suggestions for changes from that point onward. To some extent, parental behavior can be judged as being "wrong," and a great range of subtle differences of sensitivity are observable.

Recommendation: Tube weaning from temporary ENS should be performed by an experienced and specialized feeding team as early as possible when the nutritional goals have been met or when ENT is not as effective as intended. In all cases, parents must be empowered to take over feeding activities as early as possible, with generous and gentle support of the nursing and feeding team.

References

1. https://explore.notube.com/hs-fs/hub/374345/file-2406940795-pdf/our_scientific_studies/ HBeckenbachDevelopmental_impact_of_a_standardized_tube_weaning_program.pdf.   Seen on 17 Aug, 2021.
2. Khan Z, Marinschek S, Pahsini K, Scheer P, Morris N, Urlesberger B, Dunitz-Scheer M. Nutritional/growth status in a large cohort of medically fragile children receiving long-term enteral nutrition support. J Pediatr Gastroenterol Nutr. 2016;62(1):157–60. https://doi.org/10.1097/MPG.0000000000000931.
3. Sadeh-Kon T, Fradkin A, Dunitz-Scheer M, Golik-Guz T, Sarig-Klein R, David M, Weiss B, Sinai T. Long term nutritional and growth outcomes of children completing an intensive multidisciplinary tube-feeding weaning program. Clin Nutr. 2020;39(10):3153–9. https://doi.org/10.1016/j.clnu.2020.02.006.
4. Gardiner AY, Vuillermin PJ, Fuller DG. A descriptive comparison of approaches to paediatric tube weaning across five countries. Int J Speech Lang Pathol. 2017;19(2):121–7. https://doi.org/10.1080/17549507.2016.1193898.
5. Edwards S, Hyman PE, Mousa H, Bruce A, Cocjin J, Dean K, Fleming K, Romine RS, Davis AM. iKanEat: protocol for a randomized controlled trial of megestrol as a component of a pediatric tube weaning protocol. Trials. 2021;22(1):169. https://doi.org/10.1186/s13063-021-05131-w.
6. Davis AM, Bruce A, Cocjin J, Mousa H, Hyman P. Empirically supported treatments for feeding difficulties in young children. Curr Gastroenterol Rep. 2010;12(3):189–94. https://doi.org/10.1007/s11894-010-0100-9.
7. Marinschek S, Dunitz-Scheer M, Pahsini K, Geher B, Scheer P. Weaning children off enteral nutrition by netcoaching versus onsite treatment: a comparative study. J Paediatr Child Health. 2014;50(11):902–7. https://doi.org/10.1111/jpc.12662.
8. Papousek M. Communication in early infancy: an arena of intersubjective learning. Infant Behav Dev. 2007;30(2):258–66. https://doi.org/10.1016/j.infbeh.2007.02.003.

What Happens Afterward? A New Life
for Children and Parents

18

While the duration of ENS should be defined by mainly nutritional goals, the successful ending of it does not resemble the end of other medical interventions. The following chapter is based on the report of a mother and depicts the parental perspective excellently and too well not to publish it. With Jenny L.'s permission, it is presented here; her son was 5 at the time and is 12 now.

18.1 Lessons from Having a Child with a Feeding Tube

Over the days, weeks, months, and years of having a tube-fed child, I learned a lot and not just as a consequence of him being tube-fed for over 5 years. A lot of these lessons are generally applicable, but maybe tube feeding itself sometimes makes certain lessons stand out more. Have summarized our impressions here:

1. Expect the Unexpected
   A feeding tube often brings other and new problems with it. This can be anything from finding suitable clothing to dealing with severe reflux and vomiting after tube feeds while out and about. On the one hand, you learn to (usually) calmly deal with all kinds of situations that would have previously completely flustered you. On the other hand, you don't go anywhere without having a spare set of everything in case of any conceivable emergency.

2. Doctors Are Not Gods in White Coats
   After dealing with a lot of doctors and specialists, I have come to realize that medical training does not necessarily make you an expert. In fact, the best doctors are those that openly admit their own limitations to their knowledge—and then go find out more. Therefore, a gastroenterologist is not necessarily an expert on tube weaning; similarly a tube feeding team, while providing feeding tube guidelines, is also not necessarily expert on tube weaning either. Learn to question, demand answers, and not be intimidated by a medical qualification.

M. Dunitz-Scheer, P. J. Scheer, *Child-led Tube-management and Tube-weaning*,
https://doi.org/10.1007/978-3-031-09090-5_18

3. New Vocabulary

Every parent of a medically challenged or medically fragile child must learn a whole new vocabulary to cover their own child's medical history. The parent of a child with a cardiac diagnosis may speak a different language than the parent of a premature born child. Parents dealing with a feeding tube will also learn a new vocabulary and become fluent in a language that includes the different types of tube and even new terms such as tube dependency and feeding disorders in early childhood. Most people don't know that such terms or medical conditions exist—and many doctors don't know these terms either.

4. It's About More than Just Food or Hunger

Well-meant advice on getting your child to eat normally includes statements such as "Sit down to eat as a family," "He'll copy you, if he sees you eating," "Have you tried giving him anything in his mouth?", and "What about food x or y, they are really tasty." You develop a thick skin, an outward smile, and reply to such suggestions, because, let's face it, you've tried everything already. Parents are not stupid. But tube feeding and weaning is more than about hunger and types of food. It is a psychological and comprehensive process that addresses more than just hunger equals food. Once weaned, people quickly forget the earlier troubles and start urging you to only feed your child healthy foods. Meanwhile you sit there for years after the tube wean still wondering and appreciating every time your child says they are hungry, eats anything, or gets in a mess. Whether it is fast food or a healthy super food, it doesn't matter, and what matters is that your child actually EATS! And enjoys it. In fact, a lot of tube-weaned kids joyfully eat a wider variety of foods than their "non-tubie" friends and siblings.

5. Trust Your Instinct and Trust Your Child

Possibly one of the greatest lessons for any parent is to trust their own instincts when it comes to their child and in turn to trust their child. Parents are faced with a barrage of information on how to be a perfect parent, and most of the information is conflicting. Then we are faced with medical advice, family advice, feeding tube guidelines, etc., but only the parent truly knows their child. All too often a parent's concerns are ignored or overruled as being "only the parent." However only the parent spends the greatest amount of time and care with their child. Trust your instincts and don't be afraid to advocate for your family and your child.

6. It's a Child Not a Medical History

Tube weaning and eventually removing the feeding tube allowed me to become a parent rather than a constant caregiver and to see my child as a personality rather than a constant medical history. The continual weight checks and calorie counting and the tube dependency are gone, and a slice of normalcy has come into our lives. I assess my child now in terms of his general health and well-being—does he have energy? Is he in a good mood? What a change!

Outlook

Okay, the patient reader has made it all the way up to Chap. 19 and is more than ready for "the final message," the magic recipe, in any case, the real thing! If you have done your reading carefully you will expect to "know" what to do. You will have understood that every single child needs to be observed and understood from within, meaning on an emotional, motivational, functional, and developmental level, as well as taking the complexity of his or her underlying medical situation into consideration. Once we can pinpoint the child's exact stage and phase in their "journey of oralization," all that needs to be done is to reduce the tube feeds swiftly, wisely, and carefully and stay adaptive at the same time to any kind of unexpected feature needing specific attention or even change of the chosen itinerary. This seemingly simple intervention demands daily weight check on a digital scale as well as a compulsory pediatric checkup based on experience of how the child's oral skills and actual intake adjust to the changes made and supervision at least once a day, 7 days a week! The pediatrician must be sure that the child is able to start compensating its nutritional requirements by oral intake or the reduction of the tube feeds which have been changed. Special care needs to be given to urinary function and regular bowel movements, and any constipation needs to be treated, as lack of bowel movements is the most significant and common appetite killer. As the child is trying to "catch up" and supplement for the withheld tube feeds, the parents need to be supported intensively but gently to let the challenging behavioral changes on the child's part happen! This actual process of tube feeding reduction and oral catch-up can happen within 1 week or may take 2–6 weeks, but in some rare cases and depending on specific obstacles and the severity of disability, it can also take as much as 6–12 months!

What is unique about this book is that it presents a first exploration of offering professional insight into the chosen topic on a narrative and not strictly scientific level. It merges medical, nutritional, psychological, and social aspects and tries to bring the facts and perspectives together. During the process of completing this work, we have tried to present a basically straightforward matter in

M. Dunitz-Scheer, P. J. Scheer, *Child-led Tube-management and Tube-weaning*, https://doi.org/10.1007/978-3-031-09090-5_19

a simple way, but unfortunately the task has proven to be not quite as simple as it seemed at first glance. Learning to eat has been happening for thousands of years in all cultures and all over the world, with no specific social, educational, or theoretical support. Feeding one's child is considered one of the most basic drives and tasks and skills associated with normal attachment behavior, and parents, relatives, other caregivers, or even professional caretakers usually do find their own way of feeding infants and young children for the first months of their lives.

What is new today is the tube: even though tube feeding with a nutritional intention has been practiced selectively for as long as nearly 200 years, its integration as a standard medical intervention in the modern healthcare systems is quite new. When considering the efforts and means poured into the biochemical and nutritional aspects of the food industry, non-nutritional facts have not been the focus of large study designs. When an elegant thin plastic device is passed through the mouth and nose or is placed to transit from the abdominal skin surface into the stomach or jejunum, both methods carry well-calculated nutrients directly into the stomach or further. While the absorption and transit of the enteral food is well understood, we do not fully know why tube-fed children very soon "forget," stop, or do not learn to use their mouth while this is happening, independent of when the tube is placed, independent of which food is given by tube, and independent of the type of tube that is chosen.

The main flaw of this book remains to be the paucity of quotations of prospective studies on the investigated topics. As compensation, we defined distinct target issues and goals (definition, assessment, management, maintenance, oral stimulation, and weaning strategies), most of which are regarded as being clinically relevant and of academic interest but have yet to be subjected to large randomized clinical investigations.

While selected tube weaning methods performed by truly experienced teams show impressive overall success rates of around 90%, age and timing are crucial factors, as any delay will likely increase the risk of damaging side effects and decrease the child's ability to transition orally.

Another clear limitation of our book is that the presented guidelines are based exclusively on literature written in English and German and cannot reflect the clinical experience of institutions in countries outside the purview of English and German publications.

The motivation for professionals and families to change an established ENS feeding routine with any tube-fed child should be discussed critically, especially when acknowledging the impossibility of patient consent in most cases and the intrusiveness and artificiality of temporary ENS. Since the need for primary tube placement usually involved a change in mindset, the return to oral feeding after months or years of ENS can again become a highly stressful, anxiety-driven, and often underestimated challenge. The discontinuation of ENS must advocate for the child's well-being, which is decided by the involved adults, as most of the children themselves are likely not able to participate in any kind of informed consent process due to their age and developmental level.

ENS always involves an externally controlled intrusion into a patient's hunger-saturation and sleep-wake biorhythm, and the range of possible long-term consequences of ENS is not known at this point. The assumption that natural oral feeding is healthier, full of relish, and socially more appropriate must also be included in any attempt to help a child establish or return to oral feeding.

Eating development is part of a greater cultural achievement, and cooking and mealtime cultures differ widely around the world. It may well be that children transition more easily and readily to oral feeding after temporary ENS in countries with less structured and rigid mealtime routines and, possibly, fewer external recommendations concerning the timing and introduction of specific age-related nutrients. Tube placement and care is restricted to countries with high standards in medicine, and the threshold to try to feed a medically fragile child by natural means may be lower in places where ENS is not easily accessible or accessible at all.

Another intriguing aspect of tube placement and removal is the general ambiguity regarding who carries the medical responsibility of tube-related issues. This is true for any legal aspects as well as outcome of ENS once it has started. Since ENS is often treated as being an intervention involving "only food" and is structurally not considered a medical intervention in a strict sense, the immediate responsibility for handling patients on ENS surprisingly is undefined. Additionally, children receiving ENS very often are medically fragile and complex patients and are seen by several specialists. Despite the numerous specialists involved, it is possible and quite frequent that no one feels specialized enough to deal with exclusively tube-related concerns and ENS-associated side effects. This adds to the difficulty of scientific analysis, and in these situations, the tendency to make the parents primarily responsible for any symptom around ENS is common, but wrong. The family systems of tube-dependent children are stressed and exhausted. This factor makes it even more crucial to ensure the well-being of children placed on ENS and for medical professionals to understand that this state is secondary and reactive to the immediate impact of ENS. This is particularly true if the amount and severity of unintended side effects outweigh the originally intended benefits.

The "main objective of monitoring nutrition support is to ensure safety and optimal growth and to detect and treat clinical complications as quickly as possible." We hope that this paper has added some specific insight into fulfilling these demands.

We believe that the setup of online database systems for all pediatric patients receiving ENS is essential to enhance critical outcome evaluation and further research. The correlation between duration, volume, and the content of ENS and micronutrients, with the underlying medical condition, the microbiome, and possible unintended side effects that compromise the expected benefits of ENS, will need further research and investigation in multicenter studies. This is also reflected in the fact that there has only been one study on the issue of long-term growth and the general outcome of medically fragile enterally fed children with mixed diagnosis with a huge pediatric range. Any further outcome analysis has to be correlated to a wide range of comorbidities. The heterogeneous nature of the underlying medical conditions, the severity of impairment of these medically fragile patients, and the diversity of enteral feeding practices in different countries make outcome evaluations difficult and seemingly impossible. Further studies will need to fill in the gap between established best clinical evidence-based practice and results based on well-defined prospective study designs.

The future: A transnational data collection system in for children on ENS for any period longer than 3 months would enable further analysis, research, and comprehension of the long-term outcome of pediatric patients on temporary or permanent ENS. This would enable a more thoroughly detailed and structured organization and monitoring of the children and help to optimize the use of ENS, with the best possible effect and least possible risk in every case.